This book is dedicated to: my father Reginald Henson who lost his battle against chronic illness on 4 January 2000 and to my mother Barbara Henson who also lost her battle for life on 9 September 2009.

I would also like to dedicate this book to our dear friend Huw Owain Price 1980–2014 and to his wife Louise and son Henry for whom life will never be quite the same.

# Mana
# and C...

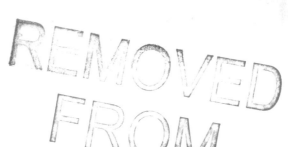

Effective management of long-term conditions is an essential part of contemporary nursing policy and practice. Systematic and evidence-based care which takes account of the expert patient and reduces unnecessary hospital admissions is vital to support those with long-term conditions/chronic diseases and those who care for them.

Reflecting recent changes in treatment, the nurse's role and the patient journey, and including additional content on rehabilitation, palliative care and non-medical prescribing, this fully updated new edition highlights the key issues in managing long-term conditions. It provides a practical and accessible guide for nurses and allied health professionals in the primary care environment and covers:

- the physical and psychosocial impact of long-term conditions
- effective case management
- self-management and the expert patient
- behavioural change strategies and motivational counselling
- telehealth and information technology
- nutritional and medication management.

Packed with helpful, clearly written information, *Managing Long-term Conditions and Chronic Illness in Primary Care* includes case studies, fact boxes and pointers for practice. It is ideal reading for pre- and post-registration nursing students taking modules on long-term conditions, and will be a valuable companion for pre-registration students on community placements.

**Judith Carrier** is a Senior Lecturer and Co-Director of Postgraduate Taught Studies at the School of Healthcare Sciences, Cardiff University. Her research and teaching interests are in evidence synthesis, evidence utilisation, primary care nursing and the management of long-term conditions, particularly diabetes. She is an active member and Director of the Wales Centre for Evidence-Based Care, a collaborating centre of the Joanna Briggs Institute, Adelaide, Australia.

# Managing Long-term Conditions and Chronic Illness in Primary Care

## A guide to good practice

Second edition

**Judith Carrier**

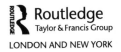 Routledge
Taylor & Francis Group

LONDON AND NEW YORK

First published 2009
by Routledge
2 Park Square, Milton Park, Abingdon, Oxon OX14 4RN

This edition published 2016
by Routledge
2 Park Square, Milton Park, Abingdon, Oxon OX14 4RN

and by Routledge
711 Third Avenue, New York, NY 10017

*Routledge is an imprint of the Taylor & Francis Group, an informa business*

*British Library Cataloguing-in-Publication Data*
A catalogue record for this book is available from the British Library

*Library of Congress Cataloging in Publication Data*
Carrier, Judith, 1960– , author.
 Managing long-term conditions and chronic illness in primary care :
 a guide to good practice / written by Judith Carrier.—Second edition.
   p. ; cm.
 Includes bibliographical references and index.
 I. Title.
 [DNLM:  1. Chronic Disease—nursing.   2. Nursing Care—methods.
 3. Case Management.   4. Long-Term Care.   5. Primary Health Care.
 WY 152.2]
 RC108
 610.73—dc23

                                        2014049455

ISBN: 978-0-415-65716-7 (hbk)
ISBN: 978-0-415-65717-4 (pbk)
ISBN: 978-0-203-07730-6 (ebk)

Typeset in Sabon
by Keystroke, Station Road, Codsall, Wolverhampton

# Contents

# Figures

# Boxes

reporting that their day-to-day activities were limited because of a health problem/disability. Since 2003/4 there has been a slight increase in adults reporting being treated for diabetes, mental illness and high blood pressure and a slight decrease for heart conditions and arthritis (WG 2013a). A report published by the Institute of Public Health in Ireland, *Making Chronic Conditions Count* (Barron et al. 2010) forecasts an increase in prevalence of a number of LTCs by 30 per cent.

Data from the QOF, through which GPs supply information in relation to chronic disease prevalence and quality indicators, allows for a more accurate picture of the prevalence of specific LTCs within the UK than self-reported data and are updated annually. At the time of publication results for England can be accessed through the Health and Social Care Information Centre (www.hscic.gov.uk/qof); this includes links to QOF data in Wales, Scotland and Northern Ireland. These do not however take into account differences between populations such as age, gender or other factors that influence prevalence or allow for analysis of co-morbidity (people with more than one condition). The most prevalent conditions covered by the QOF are hypertension, depression and asthma with prevalence of cancers, chronic kidney disease and diabetes rapidly on the increase. Not all LTCs are included on QOF registers; for example a number of musculoskeletal and neurological conditions are excluded. The impact on the NHS of caring for people with LTCs remains considerable, with some of these issues outlined in Box 1.2.

---

### Box 1.2   The impact on the NHS of caring for people with LTCs

People with LTCs are heavy users of health care resources and account for:

- 50 per cent of all GP appointments
- 64 per cent of outpatient appointments
- 70 per cent of all inpatient bed days
- 18 per cent are in receipt of state-funded social care.

People living in deprived areas are more likely to experience mental health problems alongside physical illness or disability than those in more affluent areas.

(Coulter et al. 2013)

---

Similar pictures exist in other countries. In Ireland, fewer adults overall report having an LTC, however the gradient rises steeply with age with over 50 per cent of over 65s reporting having a chronic illness or condition alongside a marked correlation between social class and self-reported health (An Roinn Slainte Department of Health 2012). In New Zealand chronic illness is the leading cause of morbidity and mortality, responsible for more than 80 per cent of deaths; this is particularly evident in Maori, Pacific peoples and those with poor socioeconomic status, chronic conditions accounting for 80 per cent of the difference between life expectancy in Maoris and non-Maori populations

(Connolly and Boyd 2011). Prevalence of chronic disease has continued to increase in Australia with nearly all people aged 65 and over reporting having one LTC, 80 per cent of these reporting having three or more conditions. Chronic diseases are cited as the major cause of death, the most common causes including cardiovascular disease, cancer, respiratory disease and diabetes (Australian Government Department of Health 2012). The focus in surveillance in Australia has been on 12 chronic conditions which are considered to pose a significant burden in terms of morbidity, mortality and health care costs, but which are open to preventative measures (see Box 1.3).

---

### Box 1.3    Twelve chronic conditions open to preventative measures

Ischaemic heart disease (also known as coronary heart disease)
Stroke
Lung cancer
Colorectal cancer
Depression
Type 2 diabetes
Arthritis
Osteoporosis
Asthma
Chronic obstructive pulmonary disease (COPD)
Chronic kidney disease
Oral disease

(Australian Institute of Health and Welfare (AIHW) 2013)

---

Chronic diseases – such as heart disease, cancer and diabetes – are the leading causes of death and disability in the USA and continue to be the most common, costly and preventable of all health problems. In 2012 about half of all adults (49.8 per cent, 117 million people) in the USA had one or more chronic health problems, with one in four adults having two or more chronic health conditions, chronic disease accounted for seven of the top ten causes of death, with heart disease and cancer accounting for nearly 48 per cent of all deaths (Centers for Disease Control and Prevention (CDCP) 2014). The majority of US health care and economic costs associated with medical conditions are related to chronic diseases and conditions. In addition to medical costs are costs associated with decreased productivity and indirect medical costs such as nursing home care (CDCP 2014).

## Policy drivers – United Kingdom

Although there is one NHS across the UK, health and social care policies vary in England, Wales, Scotland and Northern Ireland. All, however, have a similar aim,

4. Provide staff with access to the training that ensures that they have the right knowledge, skills and approach to long-term conditions care
5. Introduce a systematic and integrated multi-agency approach across community health partnerships (CHPs) to provide better, local and faster access to services for people with long-term conditions who require proactive and coordinated support
6. Strengthen the contribution that Managed Clinical/Care Networks make to the management of long-term conditions by extending their reach and ensuring full patient and carer involvement in their work
7. Adopt and sustain information systems that support registration, recall and review for people with multiple conditions, and enable effective data sharing across all relevant partners and care settings.

(Scottish Government 2009b)

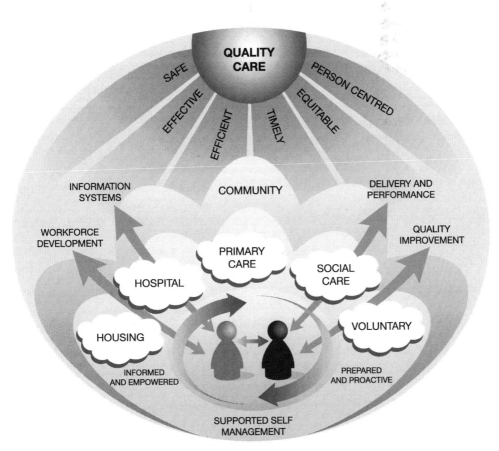

**Figure 1.3** Scotland's Mutual Care Model for Long Term Conditions

## Northern Ireland

A major initiative in Northern Ireland has been on investment in LTCs to use innovative new ways of bringing better care to people and reduce reliance on hospitals (Northern Ireland Executive 2008). New approaches to chronic disease management are being pursued using technology for remote monitoring of patients' vital signs in their homes to promote early intervention when problems arise and avoid hospital admissions. The system in Northern Ireland includes greater integration of health and social care than elsewhere in the UK. *A Healthier Future – a Twenty Year Vision for Health and Well-being in Northern Ireland* (DHSSPSNI 2005) set out Northern Ireland's vision for health and personal social service development from 2005 to 2025. The vision for chronic conditions is outlined in the following brief summary:

> Chronic conditions are a major focus of attention for health and social services, with chronic disease managed in communities, wherever possible with support from hospital services. Patients will be referred to Chronic Condition Management (CCM) programmes run in local primary and community care facilities. Seven major service-wide CCM programmes will promote chronic condition management. These include enhanced management of: diabetes, coronary heart disease, stroke recovery, arthritis and muscular-skeletal problems, chronic obstructive pulmonary disease and asthma, depression and stress management. The programmes will be tailored for people suffering from one or more chronic condition to maximise resources. Support with self-management will enable people to take greater control of their own lives, reducing severity of symptoms and improving confidence and self-efficacy.
>
> (DHSSPSNI 2005)

In 2012 DHSSPSNI published *Living with Long Term Conditions – A Policy Framework* (2012a). Its purpose was to outline a framework to help health and social care providers, including voluntary and community sectors and independent care providers, to support people with LTCs and their carers. Each chapter within the document considers a specific development area and a high level principle relevant to that area (Box 1.8).

---

### Box 1.8   *Living with Long Term Conditions –*
### *A Policy Framework* summary

1. **Working in partnership**
   The person, and the interests of the person, should be at the centre of all relationships. People, and where appropriate their carers, must be recognised as partners in the planning of services, which should be integrated and based on collaborative working across all sectors.

- Have any specific service delivery models of care been adopted in your locality?
- What system(s) have been put in place in your own practice area to ensure that the specific needs of people with LTCs are being met?
- What evaluation methods have been employed to determine the effectiveness of any approach that has been employed?

# 2 Physical, psychological and psychosocial impact of living with an LTC and social influences on health

## Overview

This section reviews the current evidence that considers the impact that the diagnosis of a long-term condition (LTC) can have on someone's life, including some of the physical, psychological and psychosocial effects of living with a LTC, both general and condition specific. Social and cultural influences on health are discussed, along with the importance of involving families and carers in care planning.

## Introduction

Living with an LTC impacts on individuals in a number of ways, ranging from increased visits to the hospital/GP and dealing with complex medical regimes, to financial difficulties and social isolation from friends and family. A British Medical Journal (BMJ 2000, p.526) editorial summed up the difference between acute and chronic disease as follows:

> With acute disease the treatment aims to return to normal. With chronic disease, the patient's life is irreversibly changed. Neither the disease nor its consequences

are static. They interact to create illness patterns requiring continuous and complex management.

Living with an LTC is not just about living with the impact on physical health; LTCs are associated with depression and other psychological impacts on health. In addition LTCs have a wider reaching social impact, affecting every part of an individual's life including family relationships, employment and everyday socialisation. Having an LTC can limit an individual's ability to go to work, school or even take care of their own day-to-day physical needs. The Department of Health (DH 2008b) note that over all ages, people with an LTC affecting their day-to-day activity are twice as likely to be out of employment compared to those without LTCs. NHS Inform, a national health information service for the public in Scotland, notes that common issues affecting many people with LTCs can include: shock; difficulty with coming to terms with their diagnosis; lack of understanding from family, friends and employers; social exclusion; fear, frustration, anger and resentment; loss of self-esteem; stress and difficulties dealing with day-to-day symptoms. Whilst these are not symptoms of mental health problems they can trigger anxiety, depression and other psychological problems (NHS Inform 2013). NHS Inform also note that 30 per cent of people with LTCs will have potential mental ill health compared with only 9 per cent of other adults.

It is not only the individual with the LTC who is affected, caring for someone with an LTC can also have an impact on health. The health and well-being of carers should be safeguarded through provision of the support required to continue in their caring role (Department of Health, Social Services and Public Safety (DHSSPSNI) 2012a). Rees et al. conducted a systematic review in 2001 which considered the impact of chronic disease on the quality of life of carers and concluded that partners who are carers also face numerous difficulties including:

- Fear of the future
- Depression and/or anxiety
- Deterioration in partner relationship and/or sex life
- Concern about suffering of patient
- Implications of the caregiving role on their own health
- Fatigue/sleep deprivation
- Social disruption – either through looking after spouse or being unwilling to attend social functions alone
- Financial difficulties – patient and/or partner unable to continue working, expense of private care and adaptations to home.

(adapted from Rees et al. 2001)

Unpaid carers, i.e. family, friends and neighbours, provide around 70 per cent of care in the community; as life expectancy increases carers may continue their caring roles for much longer periods and be caring for people with multiple and increasingly complex needs (Public Health Wales Observatory 2009).

This chapter will explore some of the physical, psychological and social impacts of living with an LTC for individuals, their families and carers.

## Physical impact

As noted in Chapter 1, LTCs cover a range of conditions including: diabetes, cardiovascular disease (CVD), which includes heart disease, stroke and other diseases of the heart and circulation such as hypertension, congestive heart failure and peripheral arterial disease (PAD), chronic kidney disease (CKD), respiratory conditions such as asthma and chronic obstructive pulmonary disease (COPD), musculoskeletal conditions such as arthritis and osteoporosis, neurological conditions such as epilepsy, multiple sclerosis, Parkinson's and motor neurone disease (MND), skin disorders such as psoriasis, genetic conditions such as cystic fibrosis and muscular dystrophy, as well as certain mental conditions such as schizophrenia and dementia. This list is merely an example of the better-known conditions and is by no means conclusive. Indeed the World Health Organisation (WHO 2013) *Global Action Plan for the Prevention and Control of Noncommunicable Diseases* notes that although the main focus of the WHO's plan is on four types of non-communicable diseases (NCDs) – cardiovascular diseases, cancer, diabetes and chronic respiratory disease – there are many other conditions of public health importance that are closely associated with the four major NCDs and these include:

1. Other NCDs (renal, endocrine, neurological, haematological, gastroenterological, hepatic, musculoskeletal, skin and oral diseases and genetic disorders).
2. Mental disorders.
3. Disabilities including blindness and deafness.
4. Violence and injuries.

The WHO (2002b) noted that physical disability or 'structural problems' including blindness or amputation are often the result of improper prevention or management of chronic conditions and this still continues to be the case. Diagnosis of an LTC is often made at a late stage of disease when long-term complications and disability are evident or acute events occur that require costly health care interventions (WHO 2010). The physical effects of all LTCs can include pain, disability and change in the condition itself that can result in hospitalisation or more intensive care requirements, in addition to the potential development of both short- and long-term complications. A King's Fund report by Goodwin et al. (2010) *Managing People with Long-term Conditions* notes that the focus on LTC management derives from a 1990s policy environment that showed that a growing proportion of inpatient activity was fuelled by people with LTCs, arguing that effective management could stabilise activity and reduce the frequent crisis and observed increases in inpatient stays associated with LTCs. Recently this picture has improved; the Wales Audit Office (2014) for example note that the positive steps that have been made to support service developments for patients with, or at risk of, chronic condition have resulted in reduced hospital admissions and a rebalance towards care provided in the community.

Whilst pain, disability and complications can be common side effects of a number of LTCs, many of the physical effects people experience are condition specific. It would be impractical to attempt to describe the physical conditions and complications associated with all LTCs. This section will instead provide an overview of some of the physical effects associated with the more prevalent LTCs mentioned previously.

## Diabetes mellitus

The prevalence of diabetes mellitus ranges worldwide, from an average 4.6 per cent of the population in the UK in 2012, to 37.5 per cent of the population in the South Pacific island of Tokelau (International Diabetes Federation (IDF) 2014). A diagnosis of diabetes is associated with significant potential short- and long-term complications (listed in Box 2.1), as well as the dietary and lifestyle changes required to achieve adequate control of the condition. For those diagnosed with type 1 diabetes, there is the additional impact of adjusting to a lifestyle regime of insulin injections and regular blood glucose monitoring. For those diagnosed with type 2 diabetes, although initial treatment may involve diet/lifestyle changes only or a combination of diet and oral hypoglycaemic medication, many people progress to eventual treatment with insulin injections.

---

## Box 2.1   Complications of diabetes mellitus

### Short-term (acute) complications

Diabetic Ketoacidosis (DKA)
Hyperosmolar Hyperglycaemic Non-ketotic coma (HONK)
Hypoglycaemia

### Long-term (chronic) complications

#### *Microvascular*

Retinopathy
Nephropathy
Neuropathy

#### *Macrovascular*

Cardiovascular disease (CVD)
Peripheral vascular/arterial disease (PVD/PAD)
Diabetic Foot (associated with PVD/PAD and/or neuropathy)

---

The short-term complications of diabetes mellitus include the life-threatening disorders of DKA and HONK, as well as hypoglycaemia. DKA is a life-threatening complication of diabetes requiring emergency medical treatment; about 20 per cent of cases are seen in undiagnosed type 1 diabetes, with the rest of cases either associated with infection, other illnesses, CVD, inadequate insulin use or unknown causes. It is much commoner in younger people, particularly females; mortality rates vary from 1–10 per cent and are linked with case mix and management expertise (Patient UK 2014a). Hyperosmolar hyperglycaemic state (HHS) or HONK is more commonly seen in older people with type 2 diabetes. It occurs through a combination of intercurrent illness, dehydration and an inability to take normal medication due to illness. Like DKA it is a potentially life-threatening condition, characterised by severe hyperglycaemia, with blood glucose levels often over 40 mmol/l and marked serum hyperosmolarity, but without evidence of severe ketosis due to the presence of basal insulin secretion. Patients normally present as extremely ill with signs of gross dehydration and require emergency medical treatment; mortality rate is 10–20 per cent (Patient UK 2014b).

Hypoglycaemia is more common, but also easier to treat, providing the person with diabetes is made aware of the symptoms and what to do. It can affect people with diabetes taking insulin and also those taking certain oral hypoglycaemic medication. Treatment is simple and involves the person taking a fast acting carbohydrate, followed up by a longer acting carbohydrate (Diabetes UK 2014). However, if left untreated it can lead to unconsciousness requiring treatment by intramuscular glucagon (given by a trained user) or intravenous glucose (given by a health professional). Some people with diabetes may suffer with problematic hypoglycaemia or hypoglycaemia unawareness (National Institute for Health and Care Excellence (NICE) 2004b). Hypoglycaemic brain damage can also occur if hypoglycaemia is not treated correctly (NICE 2004b).

The potential long-term complications of diabetes include diabetic retinopathy causing deterioration in vision which can lead to eventual loss of vision; neuropathy which can cause numerous physical effects such as erectile dysfunction (ED), muscle wasting, reduced neurological sensation, foot deformities and gastric disturbances; CKD that can progress to end stage renal failure and CVD including heart disease, stroke and PVD which can lead to limb amputation. Diabetes continues to be the leading cause of vision loss in adults of working age (20 to 65 years) in industrialised countries, the leading cause of non-traumatic limb amputation and the largest cause of kidney failure in developed countries, responsible for huge dialysis costs (IDF 2014). People with diabetes are five times more likely to develop CVD compared to those without diabetes and are at much risk of having a myocardial infarction (MI) as those who have already had a previous cardiac event. Effective management and education can reduce the risk of both short- and long-term complications.

## Cardiovascular disease (CVD)

CVD is an umbrella term for all diseases of the heart and circulation, involving coronary heart disease (CHD), cerebrovascular disease and PVD/PAD; physical effects vary dependent on the diagnosis. Risk factors for CVD include: smoking, hypertension, hyperlipidaemia, physical inactivity, being overweight or obese, having a diagnosis of diabetes and having a family history of heart disease. Physical effects of CVD range from the pain or tightness in the chest, arm, neck or jaw associated with angina, to the crushing pain, heaviness or chest tightness that can be the first sign of an MI;

long-term skin conditions can cause significant physical effects, including pain, discomfort and potential complications. *Eczema*, for example, can present as:

- Mild: with areas of dry skin and/or infrequent itching
- Moderate: with areas of dry skin, frequent itching and redness
- Severe: causing redness, with or without excoriation, extensive skin thickening, bleeding, oozing, cracking and alteration of pigmentation
- Infected: indicated by areas of weeping; crusted or pustules; fever or malaise; rapidly worsening eczema; or eczema that has failed to respond to treatment.

(CKS 2013b)

*Psoriasis*, which affects 2–3 per cent of the population of the UK, varies greatly in severity, from small, red, flaky, crusty patches that come and go, to more severe forms that may require intensive medical or nursing care. Between 10 per cent and 20 per cent of people with psoriasis develop psoriatic arthritis, which causes general tiredness, tenderness, pain and swelling over tendons, swollen fingers and toes, stiffness, pain, throbbing, swelling and tenderness in one or more joints, reduced range of movement and nail changes (The Psoriasis Association 2014). Similar to all of the LTCs, individuals suffering with long-term skin conditions need appropriate management, support and advice to help them manage their conditions and reduce physical symptoms. Psoriasis is a complex condition, unique to each individual and the physical and psychological effects of the condition should be assessed together to initiate an appropriate treatment plan (The Psoriasis Association 2014).

### Pause for reflection

Think about your own lifestyle, what would you have to change if you developed an LTC?

This section has provided an overview of some of the physical problems associated with living with an LTC. It is clear that the onset of an LTC can bring with it significant physical changes, and subsequent lifestyle adjustment requirements, in addition to an increased risk of mortality. Health care professionals through regular monitoring and review can assist people with LTCs in making these lifestyle adjustments and ensure appropriate treatment and care plans are devised and instigated to maximise health and minimise side effects, relating to both the condition and treatment. People with LTCs should also be provided with information regarding appropriate charities that can provide help and advice specific to each LTC.

## Psychological/psychosocial impact

Depression is a broad and heterogeneous diagnosis. Central to it is depressed mood and/or loss of pleasure in most activities. A chronic physical health problem can both cause and exacerbate depression: pain, functional impairment and disability associated with chronic physical health problems can greatly increase the risk of depression in people with physical illness, and depression can also exacerbate the pain and distress associated with physical illnesses and adversely affect outcomes, including shortening life expectancy.

(NICE 2009a, introduction)

Depression affects an estimated 10 per cent of the adult population. By the year 2020, it is estimated that depression will be surpassed only by heart disease in terms of the disability it causes with substantial personal, social and economic impacts (WHO 2002b). Although depression on its own is considered as an LTC, depression has also been noted as a significant co-morbidity with other LTCs and is approximately two to three times more common in a patient with a chronic physical health problem, occurring in about 20 per cent of people (NICE 2009a). As well as patients with LTCs being more likely to develop depression, it has also been suggested that people who are depressed are more likely to develop a physical LTC (Elder and Holmes 2002). Depression is frequently accompanied by anxiety symptoms but may occur on its own (NICE 2009a). Depression ranges greatly in severity, with symptoms including tearfulness, irritability, reduced sleep and appetite, pain, fatigue, lack of libido, lowered self-esteem, marked anxiety and can lead to attempts at self-harm and suicide (NICE 2009a).

Lyons et al. (2006) in their report *Long-Term Conditions and Depression*, undertaken for the Care Services Improvement Partnership (CSIP), note that depression, as cause or consequence of physical illness particularly diabetes, cardiovascular and cerebrovascular disease, may exacerbate the perceived severity of symptoms and distress and increase the utilisation of health services. Patients with cardiac disease and depression have been shown to be at increased risk of death; similarly depressed people without cardiac disease have been shown to have increased risk of cardiac mortality (NICE 2009a). Lyons et al. (2006) summarise the key issues regarding the mental health component of LTCs as shown in Box 2.2.

---

## Box 2.2   Key issues regarding the mental health component of LTCs

The mental health component of long-term conditions adversely impacts on:

- health outcomes
- disabilities
- health resource utilisation.

Medically unexplained symptoms are:

- common
- a significant cause of disability and distress
- costly.

(adapted from Lyons et al. 2006, p.13)

Certain LTCs such as stroke result in not only complex physical consequences but psychological, emotional and social sequelae which are often deep rooted (Thompson and Ryan 2008). A review of the psychosocial consequences of stroke carried out by Thompson and Ryan (2008, p.178) suggested a number of key consequences of stroke that impact on both individuals and their spouses:

- **Dependency.** Oversolicitous care of the person with stroke fostering helplessness and dependency. Decline in social interaction can jeopardise spousal relationships.
- **Loss of work.** Associated loss of income, reduced social contact and changes in lifestyle can have detrimental effects on a stroke survivor's relationship with his/her partner.
- **Fatigue.** Lowers motivation, interferes with physical functioning, work, family and social life.
- **Decline in sexual activity.** Many people experience a decline in sexual activity after a stroke. Psychological issues such as fear of a recurrent stroke, impaired self-esteem, changes in body image and a reluctance to discuss sexuality with a spouse are contributing factors.

Also noted in the review was that in a study utilising the European Brain Injury Questionnaire, depressive mood, loneliness, cognitive difficulties and lack of autonomy were the most frequent problems reported by stroke survivors.

Depression and disability have been noted as predictors of mortality in patients discharged from hospital following acute exacerbations of COPD (Halpin 2008). Links between COPD, depression and anxiety have been well documented (British Lung Foundation 2014) with the physical effects of living with lung disease, such as tiredness, difficulty in sleeping and eating, self-consciousness about coughing or needing to use oxygen and an inability to participate in activities previously enjoyed resulting in depression. Many people with COPD become anxious due to not feeling in control of their health. The British Lung Foundation (2014) provides advice and guidance to encourage people with COPD who are feeling anxious and/or depressed to seek help and support.

---

## Pause for reflection

What services are you aware of that you could refer someone to who is suffering with anxiety and depression related to an LTC?

---

Numerous other LTCs are also linked with increased incidence of depression. Depression is thought to affect about half of all people with Parkinson's disease (National Collaborating Centre for Chronic Conditions (NCC-CC) 2006). Mayor (2007) makes the point that the diagnosis of mild depression can be difficult to make in Parkinson's because of the overlapping of motor symptoms with features of clinical depression. She also notes that depression is the single most important predictor of quality in life in Parkinson's disease, can impair efforts to control symptoms and cause tension with carers. It has also been shown that depression is three times more likely in patients suffering from rheumatoid arthritis (Sheehy et al. 2006). Other physical conditions where depression is likely include: dementia, alcoholism and drug abuse and chronic pain.

In the UK, the GMS contract has identified patients with CHD and diabetes as priority for screening, practices undertaking National Enhanced Service are obliged to recognise depression at an early stage in any patient and NICE (2009a) recommends that those with a past history of depression or who have a chronic physical illness associated with functional impairment should be asked the following two questions:

- During the last month, have you been feeling down, depressed or hopeless?
- During the last month, have you often been bothered by having little interest or pleasure in doing things?

If a patient with a chronic physical illness answers 'yes' to either question, the following three questions should be asked:

During the last month, have you often been bothered by:

- Feelings of worthlessness?
- Poor concentration?
- Thoughts of death?

A positive answer to either of the first two questions should be followed up with referral to a GP for further screening, using one of three validated screening tools: the Patient Health Questionnaire, Hospital Anxiety and Depression Scale or the Beck Depression Inventory, Second Edition. An appropriate treatment plan should then be put into place if indicated.

This section has provided a brief overview of some of the potential psychological impact on health for people with LTCs. Living with an LTC is clearly not just about living with the physical effects of illness. Health care providers should be aware of the signs and symptoms of depression and anxiety, utilise suitable screening tools and instigate appropriate programmes of care in conjunction with mental health professionals to ensure people with LTCs receive appropriate treatment and support.

## Social influences on health

It is well established that health status is largely determined by a person's social environment and vice versa. The WHO (2010) note that morbidity and mortality from LTCs is greater in low and middle income countries. Policy documents in recent decades have shifted the emphasis from a focus on individual responsibility for health to a more holistic approach that includes socio-economic, environmental and cultural

# 3 | Case management and disease-specific care management

## Overview

The current policy emphasis continues to be on moving patients out of acute care settings and providing care in the community. For patients with long-term conditions (LTCs) it has long been accepted that care should be provided in the primary care/community setting with a firm emphasis on self-care. People with LTCs use disproportionately more primary and secondary care services, a pattern set to increase with an ageing population. The role of the district nurse is currently under scrutiny with many areas adopting the community matron role who manages a case load and works closely with patients to prevent unnecessary hospital admission. This chapter will explore the principles behind case management and disease-specific care management including new and existing nursing roles and the importance of multi-disciplinary team involvement.

## Introduction

In Chapter 1 the guiding strategic and theoretical frameworks and policies relating to the care of individuals with LTCs were introduced. The aim of this chapter is to discuss in further detail the principles behind case management and disease-specific care management. Existing nursing roles such as district nursing and practice nursing in meeting the needs of people with LTCs will be reviewed, in addition to the community matron/advanced primary nurse role. The importance of adopting a team approach to care will also be discussed, appreciating the contribution made by numerous health care professionals in meeting the LTC care agenda.

The US Kaiser Permanente triangle of care management on which a number of LTC models have been based, including the Department of Health (DH 2005b) NHS and

Social Care Long Term Conditions model which has more recently been superseded by the House of Care model (Coulter et al. 2013), outlines the three-tier triangle approach, stratifying patients in order to match them to appropriate packages of care. This three-tier approach involves:

> Level 3: Case management – requires the identification of the very high intensity users of unplanned secondary care. Care for these patients is to be managed using a community matron or other professional using a case management approach, to anticipate, coordinate and join up health and social care.
> Level 2: Disease-specific care management – This involves providing people who have a complex single need or multiple conditions with responsive, specialist services using multi-disciplinary teams and disease-specific protocols and pathways, such as the National Service Frameworks and Quality and Outcomes Framework.
> Level 1: Supported self-care – collaboratively helping individuals and their carers to develop the knowledge, skills and confidence to care for themselves and their condition effectively.
>
> (DH 2005b)

The supported self-care/self-management approach to care will be discussed in Chapter 4. This chapter will concentrate on reviewing existing and new methods of care, in addition to the nursing and health care roles that contribute to them, at levels 2 and 3: case management and disease-specific care management.

## Case management

### Definition and models

The term 'case management' originates from the USA where it was developed, with its roots in social care, as a method of 'delivering holistic individualized care, tailored to the needs of people with complex health and social care problems' (Hutt et al. 2004, p.6). Initially instigated in the 1950s to provide care to patients with severe mental health problems, it was expanded for use with older people with complex health and social care needs, to both contain health care costs and coordinate services to reduce the need for institutional care (Drennan and Goodman 2004; Hutt et al. 2004). Definitions of case management include 'the process of planning, coordinating, managing and reviewing the care of an individual, with the aim being: to develop cost-effective and efficient ways of coordinating services in order to improve quality of life' (Hutt et al. 2004, p.6). Reviewing types of case management approaches, Drennan and Goodman (2004) note that two types of case manager role can be adopted: the brokerage model (similar to the UK social worker model), where case managers hold the budget to finance user care packages, and the key worker extension model, which is closer to the approach historically used by district nurses in the UK, where the case manager both provides and coordinates services for the user. Rather than being a single intervention, case management refers to a wider package of care (Ross et al. 2011).

Within the UK, England piloted the US nurse-led Evercare model, introduced in 2003 in nine Primary Care Trusts (PCTs), with appointment of Advanced Primary Nurses (APNs), also referred to as community matrons, taking on the case management role. Apart from Evercare, other US service models, developed by Pfizer and Kaiser Permanente, were also piloted in areas of the UK (see Chapter 1 for descriptions of these models). These models were by no means universal throughout the four countries of the UK, however. Wales for example developed different approaches in each locality, adopting a variety of diverse methods to take the practical aspects of the LTC management agenda forwards. This included development of LTC teams who supported practice nurses and GPs through provision of educational updates, or who worked with primary health care teams (PHCTs) to assist them with managing more complex patients.

## Community matrons

A community matron is described in the NHS plan (DH 2004b) as: 'An individual who is experienced, skilled and uses case management techniques with patients who make high use of health care services, with the ultimate aim of remaining at home longer with more choice about their health care'. The community matron/APN is expected to be an experienced nurse, already working in the NHS, who has a wide range of competencies. These include high level assessment and clinical skills to meet physical, mental and social care needs; an ability to identify high risk patients; lead complex care coordination, including liaising and synchronising inputs from other agencies; review and prescribe medications; support self-care and independence and be highly visible to patients, their families and carers and seen as being in charge of their care (DH 2005a). They manage the care of people with one or more LTCs, or who have a complex mix of medical and social problems and are intensive users of health care services, including frequent admissions to hospital. The intention behind the community matron role was that they would provide a more holistic approach to care, overseeing a caseload of up to 80 patients and coordinating health and social care provision with the overall aim of promoting maximum function, independence and improved quality of life. The role itself offers autonomy and independence to influence service delivery and maintain clinical credibility, whilst remaining closely involved with patient care.

It is important to note at this stage that nurses working in a range of roles in primary care, particularly district nurses, have always made significant contributions to the care of people with LTCs, specifically the elderly population, using case management techniques (Drennan and Goodman 2004). Indeed following the evaluation of the initial Evercare pilot sites in England, While (2007) commented that the pilot programmes had made little significant impact on overall health care outcomes, including emergency admissions and bed days, and that community matrons cannot substitute for the district nursing workforce, whose service needs to be revitalised and retooled.

Worldwide similar approaches have been adopted. Australia's National Chronic Disease Strategy (National Health Priority Action Council (NHPAC) 2006) sets out a three stage triangular approach to care, similar to the UK's (see Figure 3.1).

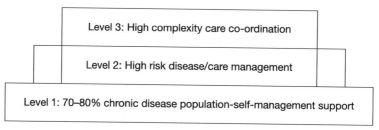

**Figure 3.1** Australia's National Chronic Disease Strategy
Source: NHPAC (2006)

Services in Australia are being developed to improve care coordination for all those with LTCs, with plans to provide integration and continuity of prevention and care, through the use of care coordinators, to ensure that multi-disciplinary care plans are carried through and regularly reviewed. Access to appropriate services is seen as a priority, particularly for Aboriginal and Torres Strait Islander peoples, rural and remote communities and other under serviced population groups (NHPAC 2006). New Zealand also has an LTCs framework (Capital and Coast District Health Board 2008; South Canterbury District Health Board 2009).

## Effectiveness of case management

A King's Fund report (Hutt et al. 2004) examined the effectiveness of case management drawing on studies mainly from the USA but also from Canada, Italy, Denmark and Scotland. The review focused particularly on the transferability of these models to the UK and identified a number of important issues. These included the variability of economic and regulatory environments between countries that can make it harder to reproduce patterns of utilisation and cost savings reported in other countries. Second they noted that the differences in training and skills of the staff providing case management raised questions about the feasibility of transferring findings from the USA to the UK NHS, with many US nurse case managers trained to Master's level. Third they noted that patient selection techniques are imprecise and do not always predict who may benefit most from case management. In addition they emphasised that components of case management could duplicate other services offered by the NHS such as hospital outreach and community-based services. Overall the review concluded that there is limited evidence regarding the most effective types of case management. Where case management is being implemented local NHS providers need to be clear about the needs of the population at whom it is aimed; discuss whether existing services can be adapted; develop case management in close collaboration with social care providers; ensure that adequate systems are in place for those with less severe illness; and evaluate initiatives in terms of both their impact on the health service and patient satisfaction (Hutt et al. 2004). A more recent King's Fund report (Goodwin et al. 2010) further suggests that case management is not always implemented in a cost effective way or to the benefit of patients and carers. The report concludes that case management programmes have significant potential to deliver cost savings and better care for patients, but must be well designed, involve appropriately trained professionals and be embedded in a system that supports and values integrated and coordinated care. They emphasise that case management works well when at risk patients are clearly identified and specialty trained nurses who assess the patient and carer needs and co-design an action plan are integrated into primary care practices.

The final report of the evaluation of Evercare pilot sites in the UK (Boaden et al. 2006) indicated a contradiction between the qualitative and quantitative findings. The qualitative findings suggested that both patients and carers experienced a high level of satisfaction with the service. They particularly valued the psychological support, the rapid response in times of crisis and the ability of the APNs to monitor medications, organise prescriptions, explain LTCs, investigations and treatments and provide advocacy for patients. The APNs reported many examples when they had altered medication and coordinated care to avoid hospital admissions, improve quality of life and reduce fragmentation of services. However the quantitative evaluation showed no significant effect on emergency admissions, emergency bed days or mortality, both for the high-risk groups and the general over 65 population. The report concluded that Evercare provided a workable model of case management, which was popular with APNs, patients and carers. It also noted that adoption of this system provided patients and carers with frequency of contact, regular monitoring and knowledge of referral procedures; options that had not previously been provided. However no overall evidence of systematic redesign of care was identified and it was noted that this would need to be addressed in future if hospital admissions were to be reduced.

### Pause for reflection

Has case management been introduced in your area, has it had an impact on overall health outcomes? If you are a case manager what educational preparation did you receive for the role, did you feel adequately prepared?

## Practicalities of case management

If a case management strategy is to be adopted identification of suitable patients/clients is essential. In order to identify which patients/clients would be most suitable for case management, those who present with the most complex conditions and are considered vulnerable, or at risk of hospitalisation, or at risk of requiring institutionalised care, need to be identified by the appropriate health and social care organisation (DH 2005b). In the UK a number of software tools have been developed that can assist with this process. Criteria for selection include the following:

- Number of hospital admissions and lengths of stay
- Co-morbidity (number of medical and other problems that a patient may have)

- Number of medications a patient is prescribed
- Number of GP consultations
- Other high risk factors (such as living alone/unsupported).

(adapted from DH 2005b)

Additional criteria used in the Evercare pilots included:

- Recent exacerbation or decompensation of chronic illness
- Recent falls (>2 falls in 2 months)
- Recent bereavement and at risk of medical decline
- Cognitively impaired, living alone, medically unstable and high intensity social service package.

(DH 2005b, p.16)

Drennan and Goodman (2004) suggest that case management has the following core activities at individual patient level (Box 3.1).

---

## Box 3.1   Core activities at individual patient level

- Identification of individuals likely to benefit from case management
- Assessment of the individual's problems and need for services
- Care planning of activities and services to address the agreed needs
- Coordination and referral to implement the care plan
- Regular review, monitoring and consequent adaptation of the care plan.

(Drennan and Goodman 2004, p.527)

---

Hutt et al. (2004) note that case management can be used for a variety of reasons. Regardless of selection criteria assessment should be a key component, with the focus varying from clinical assessment, controlling access to services and provision and coordination of different services. They further state that although the focus of nurse led case management is on clinical needs, minimising symptoms and reducing hospitalisation, nurse case managers play a key role in coordinating services from other health and social care providers. Ross et al. (2011) add that the following core components are particularly important in case management programmes: case-finding; assessment; care planning; care coordination; case closure (in a time-limited intervention). The assessment stage, in particular, should aim to identify the individual's clinical and social needs, as well as the health and well-being of any carers. Care planning is considered to be at the heart of any case management programme, bringing together individual circumstances with health and social care needs to create a plan that matches needs with service provision (Ross et al. 2011). A study undertaken by Reeves et al. (2014), however, notes that the use of written care plans in patients with LTCs in primary care is uncommon and variable among UK primary care practices and that more proactive efforts at implementation are required before their efficacy can be determined.

The overall aim of case management is to provide a holistic health and social package of care to meet the needs of the most vulnerable patients, with the most complex conditions, who have often not previously been actively managed by the whole care system.

## Disease-specific care management

The intention of the National Service Frameworks (NSFs) was to provide a structured evidence-based framework for all health care professionals and organisations to ensure equity of care and responsive specialist services for people with LTCs. NSFs tended to concentrate on condition specific areas, although broader NSFs, such as those for older people and children, look at the specific needs of groups, rather than conditions. For people with more unstable LTCs who do not necessarily require a case management approach, but do require more frequent intervention or specialist support, evidence-based guidelines (Chapter 9) can assist PHCTs in developing appropriate referral criteria and systems to ensure that this help is readily available. Specialist nurses, in areas such as diabetes or epilepsy, are an invaluable source of expertise to provide additional help and guidance. People needing more specialist input and support should be identified through the process of regular review (Chapter 8). Referral criteria derived from NSFs and evidence-based guidelines can then be built into an appropriate practice protocol or multi-disciplinary care pathway to ensure prompt referral and specialist support. DH (2005b) suggests a number of key actions to improve disease-specific care management (see Box 3.2).

---

### Box 3.2    Key actions to improve disease-specific care management

- Examination of current delivery of disease management
- Establishment of multi-disciplinary professional teams with specialist support to manage care across all settings
- Identification and pro-active management of those with LTCs using agreed standards and protocols
- Use of prompts and reminders (such as text messaging) to recall patients
- Regular review and support of those with LTCs
- Use of NSFs and quality indicators to provide a detailed approach to care.

(adapted from DH 2005b)

---

### Pause for reflection

How do you differentiate between those needing disease-specific care management and those requiring case management?

## Role of the district nurse in the management of people with LTCs

DH policies set out a clear strategy to develop sustainable, inclusive and equal health care for every individual to access a suitable health professional based on individual need (DH 2004b). The publication of the NSF for LTCs (DH 2005c) (although built upon the specific needs of those with long-term neurological conditions, it is applicable to all those with LTCs) further strengthens the need for person-centred care and collaborative approaches between health and social care to ensure people can be supported at home. *2020 Vision* (Queen's Nursing Institute (QNI) 2009) reviewed the role of the district nurse (DN) in ensuring services are developed to keep people at home where they want to be. DNs aim to build therapeutic relationships and strive to promote coping and independence, both practically and psychologically. Indeed Wilson (2005) noted that a number of the 11 quality requirements set out in the NSF are extremely pertinent to district nursing. These include:

- Provision of a person-centred service through integrated assessment and care-planning and provision of information, education, advice and support (QR1).
- Community rehabilitation and support, emphasising that rehabilitation in the home is cost-effective, reduces restrictions related to daily living and improves individual well-being (QR5).
- Providing personal care and support, with people able to exercise choice over where they wish to live (QR8).
- Palliative care, a role well established by district nurses (QR9).

The NSF for older people (Welsh Government (WG) 2006) identified that social health and care needs, including for those with LTCs, should be managed effectively within the community in order to avoid inappropriate admissions to hospital. This requires holistic assessment to ensure prompt identification of problems, which DNs undertake on a daily basis within their role.

DNs, as members of the PHCT, deliver care in a range of settings and are well placed to deliver health education, health promotion, holistic assessment and management of people with LTCs. The advantages for patients are flexible services to meet their individual needs, ensuring continuity of care with the opportunity to be supported within the home. There are however inherent problems with a nursing service that is autonomous but also highly dependent on other participants within the PHCT. Whilst being responsive to the demand the DN must also be proactive in managing LTC. The integration with other teams is becoming a huge driver for the traditional DN service. *Visions and Values* (QNI 2006) identified that patients with LTCs experience fewer exacerbations of their conditions and consequently fewer hospital admissions, if DNs manage their care. Historically DNs have always managed patients with LTCs; however this has often been in an ad hoc manner, rather than the structured case management approach advocated by the community matron/APN role. Wilson (2005) notes that DNs were probably most enabled to deliver the holistic approach suggested by today's policies before the imposition of the clear boundaries between health and social care needs formed in the early 1990s.

The main focus of the DN has been caring for people who are house bound. Many of these people, who are often elderly, have significant co-morbidities or have been diagnosed with more than one LTC. Coordinating the care for this group of patients supports the case management model of care (DH 2007a; Ross et al. 2011). The difference being that for these patients their preliminary contact with the district nursing service may be for an unrelated problem and it is only during the initial assessment process that problems are identified. Community matrons are expected to actively seek out people who would benefit from a case management approach using appropriate data. *2020 Vision Five Years On* (QNI 2014) concluded that one of the skills that DNs consistently demonstrated was their ability to conduct holistic assessments, which is essential in order to manage patients with LTCs. Effective assessment ensures that the patient is provided with evidence-based care and is an essential requirement of all members of the district nursing team. Older people often have complex needs that change rapidly. To ensure their safe management within the home environment requires development and delivery of individual care plans. DNs use a broad approach towards assessment, reassessing patients at each visit, acknowledging their changing needs and referring to other health care professionals where necessary. Advanced health assessment skills are also one of the main requirements for the community matron role, along with expert clinical skills, the key difference appearing to be in the advanced educational preparation recommended to carry out the community matron role.

The introduction of the General Medical Services (GMS) contract (British Medical Association (BMA)/NHS Confederation 2003) enabled DNs working within the PHCT to have a clearer focus when providing care to this, sometimes vulnerable, group of patients. Providing annual reviews for patients within their own homes is now commonplace ensuring a more equitable health care service. Research supports that hospital admissions are prevented by the intervention of a DN (Bernabei et al. 1998; Gagnon 1999). It can be established that care is less fragmented as DNs are able to signpost patients to the most appropriate services. DH (2006) discuss the importance of supporting and caring for people in their home environment, rather than in secondary care, particularly those over 65 and those with an LTC. They also stress the need to work more closely with social services, to support this group of people to allow them to remain at home. Of all the PHCT the DN will have key working knowledge of the social service network within their local area of practice and would therefore seem to be the person most able to organise care. It is often the most 'sick' patients who are visited by the DN when an exacerbation of their condition makes it impossible for them to attend the GP surgery. Many areas across the UK have seen the development of intermediate care services. These multi-professional services aim to deliver short intensive episodes of care with the main aim to avoid admission to secondary care. Some of these will be within district nursing teams using a virtual ward environment. This enables known patients with an exacerbation of their LTC to be reviewed by the team on a daily basis supporting them with both medical and social input to remain at home.

It would be fair to conclude that although recognised as experts in case management of highly complex patients with LTCs, DNs run the risk of losing out on this element of their role if they fail to be responsive to policy initiatives. Recent years have seen health policies developed, which although not directed at district nursing services have undoubtedly had a huge impact on their work and how they deliver care. DNs are faced with a challenge of self-perception, they should now see themselves as impressively adapted to professional and organisational change and politically influential as the policy spot light is clearly on improved and systematic management of LTCs.[1]

## Role of the practice nurse in the management of people with LTCs

In the UK the DH (1990) GP contract laid the foundations for moving primary care services away from a curative, illness led service to that of a preventative health promotion led service. GPs, through a system of financial reimbursement, were encouraged to promote health as well as treat illness, by providing services such as well person health checks and chronic disease management clinics. In order to provide these services GPs employed more practice nurses.

The rise of the clinical governance agenda (DH 1998) put an increasing emphasis not only on the provision of evidence-based care, but also on procedures such as audit in order to monitor both the quality of the care provided to patients and the quality of the organisational set up providing this care. In the primary care setting practice nurses took on much of the responsibility for providing this quality care, developing their skills and knowledge accordingly. As a profession general practice nursing evolved rapidly, with the number of full time equivalent (FTE) practice nurses in England increasing by 42 per cent from 9,745 to 13,793 between 1995 and 2005, with almost 25,000 practice nurses estimated to be working in the UK by 2005 (Royal College of General Practitioners (RCGP) 2007). Whilst the numbers declined between 2006 and 2010 practice nurse consultations have continued to rise, doubling in number between 1996 and 2009 (Centre for Workforce Intelligence (CfWI) 2012), which the report notes could be a response to the reported increase in the number, length and complexity of consultations, or alternatively may have enabled the additional required consultations to take place. The importance of strategic and systematic care of patients with LTCs, which began with the 1990 GP contract, including the 3 Rs, registration, regular recall and review (DH 2005b), was further emphasised with the publication of NSFs, the first of which to be introduced in the UK was the NSF for Coronary Heart Disease (CHD) (DH 2000a). Practice nurses quickly rose to the challenge of providing this care. By this time they had clearly demonstrated their ability to deliver effective management and strategies for people with LTCs, specifically in relation to asthma, chronic obstructive pulmonary disease (COPD), diabetes, hypertension and CHD. The GMS contract (BMA/NHS Confederation 2003), implemented in 2004, created a further expansion of the role with practice nurses progressively taking on the responsibility of meeting the demands of the Quality and Outcomes Framework (QOF) outlined in Chapter 1. The contract was seen as part of a programme of health service modernisation, with nurses seen as key players in delivering the agenda (McDonald et al. 2009). *Liberating the Talents* (DH 2002b) and the subsequent Welsh Government white paper *Setting the Direction* (WG 2010) set the context for the shifting of services from hospital to primary care settings and paved the way for primary care nurses to be given greater freedom to innovate and make decisions about the services and care they provide. At a micro level of care, McDonald et al. (2009) suggest that the impact of the GMS contract has intensified practice nurse workloads with the responsibility of meeting contract targets. Additionally it has realigned their role from one of task orientation to one of first contact care, particularly in the management of chronic disease, a process that had its origins in the 1990 GP contract and has continued to be influenced by both NHS organisational restructure and subsequent changes brought on by the GMS contract (McDonald et al. 2009).

The role of the practice nurse in regard to caring for those with LTCs includes identification, diagnosis, monitoring and management in the primary care environment:

- Identify patients for screening
- Undertake diagnostic tests, for example spirometry
- Contribute to the updating of LTC registers through accurate record keeping
- Work within evidence-based practice protocols to provide programmes of care including annual review, initial and ongoing education and preventative advice
- Review medication, assess adherence and develop concordance
- Prescribe medication as appropriate (having undertaken a recognised prescribing qualification)
- Provide support and advice for patients and their carers
- Provide advice relating to voluntary, community and patient organisations, e.g. Diabetes UK, as appropriate
- Refer to local educational programmes such as Expert
- Refer to other health and social care professionals as necessary.

Practice nurses therefore play a significant role in the management of people with LTCs in relation to both disease-specific care management and in supporting people to self-care. It is not just in the UK that practice nurses are seen as key providers in caring for patients with LTCs. Although the US health care system has not adopted the role, in other countries such as parts of Europe, Australia and New Zealand practice nurses carry out a similar role to that in the UK.

## Role of the multi-disciplinary team in the management of people with LTCs

In addition to identified nursing roles, people with LTCs may be seen by many different health and social care professionals. Coulter et al. (2013) note that to build the 'House of Care' requires involvement of a wide variety of organisations, professional groups and individuals working together in a coordinated manner using pooled budgets, shared data and learning together to deliver holistic, coordinated, person-centred care.

Occupational therapists, for example, play an important role in working with people with LTCs focusing on:

- How they can enable clients to function at an optimal level, despite impairments
- How activities which the person needs or wants to do can be modified or adapted to make them easier
- How clients feel about themselves and their ability to tackle problems
- How the physical and social environment can be altered so that restrictions are reduced.

(British Association of Occupational Therapists and
College of Occupational Therapists 2014)

In order for care to be effective, people with LTCs need to be able to access multi-professional teams based in primary or community care, who can provide them with specialist advice tailored to individual need; this should be accompanied by a move away from a reactive disease fragmented focus of care towards an approach that is pro-active, holistic and preventative (Coulter et al. 2013). Goodwin et al. (2010) make the point that to improve the quality of care in conditions such as arthritis, for example, practice nurses and GPs should make referral to a multi-disciplinary team as needed, such as physiotherapists, occupational therapists or surgeons; they should also discuss the options available to patients and support them in making decisions. For conditions such as dementia, individuals are likely to be in contact with a number of different health care professionals, social care providers and support services and GPs and practice nurses need to work in partnership with colleagues, sharing and seeking information (Goodwin et al. 2010).

The Royal Pharmaceutical Society of Great Britain and the BMA (2000) produced a report on team working in primary care. The review of the research demonstrated that benefits of teamwork could be classified as: a more responsive and patient-centred service and a more clinically and/or cost effective service which provided more satisfying team roles and career paths for health care professionals. Their recommendations in relation to teams and team members are summarised in Box 3.3.

---

### Box 3.3   Teams and team members

The team should:

- Recognise and include the patient, carer or their representative as an essential member of the primary health care team
- Establish a common, agreed purpose
- Agree set objectives and monitor progress towards them. Involve all team members in decision making and delivery of agreed objectives

- Agree team working conditions, including process for resolving conflict
- Ensure each team member understands and acknowledges the skills and knowledge of others
- Pay particular attention to communication, using technology to assist
- Ensure the practice population understand and accept the way the team works
- Select the leader for his/her leadership skills, not by hierarchy, status or availability. Include all relevant professions in the team
- Promote teamwork across heath and social care
- Evaluate team working initiatives and develop practice base on sound evidence
- Ensure sharing of patient information is in accordance with legal and professional requirements.

(adapted from Royal Pharmaceutical Society/BMA 2000, p.7)

## Examples of effective multi-disciplinary teams

A number of systematic reviews and research studies have evaluated the use of multi-disciplinary teams in contributing to the care of people with LTCs. These include a review by McAlister et al. (2004), which concluded that multi-disciplinary teams were cost effective and reduced hospital admission and overall mortality in patients with heart failure. Jackson et al. (2005) reviewed the care of over 82,000 patients with diabetes in 177 clinics and noted that weekly multi-disciplinary team meetings, special teams or protocols for clinical issues were amongst a list of factors that contributed to improved glycaemic control. The Leeds Young Adult Team provides multi-disciplinary input (physiotherapy, occupational therapy, speech and language therapy and psychology with access to contraceptive and sexual health service, social worker and consultant in rehabilitation medicine) to young adults (16–25 years) with a physical impairment. The team focuses on each individual's needs and provides information, support and treatment to enable each young person to live the kind of life they choose to lead. A retrospective cohort study of the effectiveness of this approach to care found that it produced better results at no extra cost compared to an ad hoc approach (Bent et al. 2000). DH (2005b) outline a number of examples where collaborative working has enhanced patient care. One example provided is that of a helpdesk set up in an ambulance dispatch centre to alert GPs to patients who have contacted the service regarding exacerbation of their condition, but who weren't admitted to hospital. This ensures that the GP can closely monitor those patients and avoid potential emergency admissions in the future.

In order for a multi-disciplinary team to be effective, roles and boundaries need to be apparent, with each team member aware of their role and the role of others. Boundaries can sometimes be blurred, so transparent referral criteria need to be established, with clear channels of communication open to all team members. Protocols can provide an effective way of defining the role of each team member, preventing both omissions and duplication of care. Service users should also have the opportunity to be involved in discussions and decisions made about their care. A multi-disciplinary team involved in the care of a patient with diabetes may include:

- Practice nurse and/or diabetes specialist nurse
- DN
- Diabetologist and/or GP
- Dietitian
- Podiatrist
- Optician/ophthalmologist
- Pharmacist
- Consultant from other medical specialty, e.g. renal, cardiology, vascular.

In order that the patient/client receives optimal care all decisions should be communicated to those involved in the care. Advances in information technology (see Chapter 6), with instant access to results and patient records, for all members of the team, can enhance the care provided. Specialist nurses can often provide the expertise and support that a patient requires, liaising with appropriate services and advising patients on suitable options. Multi-disciplinary teams can both contribute to and improve the proactive care provided to patients/clients with LTCs. Evidence-based care pathways and local protocols should guide health and social care professionals in delivering appropriate packages of care.

## Conclusion

Providing appropriate care for people with LTCs, particularly at levels 2 and 3: case management and disease-specific care management (DH 2005b; NHPAC 2006; Ross et al. 2011), can be complex and often involves a number of different health and social care professionals. Whatever type of approach or model of care is adopted, the key to successful management includes regular and systematic review, adequate communication and referral criteria between all team members, including the patient/client and carer and appropriate systems in place to support patients/clients in both times of stability and during exacerbations.

### Key points

- The majority of patients with LTCs are able to self-care but adequate systems need to be put into place to provide case management and disease-specific care management programmes for those patients/clients with more complex needs.

study including primary care staff, Kennedy et al. (2014) found limited evidence of the collaborative partnerships between patients and practitioners required for effective self-management support. They argue that the organisational priorities of general practice in the UK means that the work required to implement self-management support has not been given the priority it requires; this has been hindered by the task driven nature of nurses' routines and a lack of motivation by some nurses to engage with self-management support activities due to an underlying scepticism of the will of patients to take adequate responsibility for their health.

## Examples of patient directed interventions

### Problem-solving interventions

Bodenheimer et al. (2002) emphasise that whereas traditional patient education offers information and technical skills, self-management education teaches problem-solving skills. Their review of evidence from controlled clinical trials suggests that:

1. Programmes teaching self-management skills are more effective than information-only patient education in improving clinical outcomes.
2. In some circumstances, self-management education improves outcomes and can reduce costs for arthritis and probably for adult asthma patients.
3. In initial studies, a self-management education programme bringing together patients with a variety of chronic conditions may improve outcomes and reduce costs.

A systematic review of the literature on problem-solving interventions and its associations with diabetes self-management and control (Hill-Briggs and Gemmell 2007) concluded that cross-sectional studies in adults, but not children/adolescents, provided consistent evidence of associations between problem solving and HbA1c level (a key indicator of glycaemic control in diabetes). They defined problem solving as 'a multidimensional construct encompassing verbal reasoning/rational problem solving, quantitative problem solving, and coping'. Despite methodological limitations 25 per cent of problem-solving intervention studies with children/adolescents and 50 per cent of interventions with adults reported improvement in HbA1c, although effect on behavioural and psychosocial outcomes was varied. Most intervention studies reported an improvement in behaviours, most commonly global adherence in children/adolescents and dietary behaviour in adults. A 2012 update of this review (Fitzpatrick et al.) included a further 24 studies that reported a problem-solving intervention or used problem solving as an intervention component for diabetes self-management training and disease control. Despite significant variability amongst the approaches to problem-solving use in patient education, 36 per cent of adult problem-solving interventions and 42 per cent of children/adolescent problem-solving interventions demonstrated significant improvement in HbA1c, alongside some promising positive effects on psychosocial outcomes amongst adults and children/adolescents, including communication. It is recommended that future intervention studies should clearly identify what constitutes problem-solving training, to determine exactly which factors influence outcomes.

## Action plans

Handley et al. (2006) define an action plan as 'an agreement between clinician and patient that the patient will make a specific behaviour change'. Handley et al.'s (2006) descriptive study based in a primary care setting involved 228 patients across eight primary care sites. Fifty-three per cent of patients reported making a behaviour change based on the action plan, suggesting that action plans may be a useful strategy to encourage behaviour change for patients seen in primary care.

Action plans have been noted as successful in assisting patients in self-management of specific conditions, asthma in particular. Most of the available evidence about self-management treatment plans focuses on asthma and COPD, although there is some evidence emerging about other conditions (de Silva 2011). A systematic review by Powell and Gibson (2002) concluded that optimisation of asthma control by self-adjustment of medications with the aid of a written action plan was equivalent to that by regular medical review. Individualised written action plans based on peak expiratory flow (PEF) measurements, were equivalent to action plans based on symptoms. Toelle and Ram (2004) in a later review however suggested that there is not enough evidence to show that personalised, written self-management plans for asthma, as the sole intervention, improve health outcomes. They conclude that to change asthma management behaviour and improve health outcomes requires a coordinated approach of self-management education, regular review and a written action plan.

In other conditions, for example COPD, the effectiveness of action plans used as a singular intervention is ineffective. Turnock et al.'s (2005) systematic review concluded that although there is evidence that action plans aid people with COPD in recognising and reacting appropriately to an exacerbation of their symptoms via the self-initiation of antibiotics or steroids, there was no evidence of significant effects on health care utilisation, health-related quality of life, lung function, functional capacity, symptom scores, mortality, anxiety or depression. The 2010 update of this review (Walters et al.) concluded that the practice of giving individual action plans and limited self-management education for patients with COPD exacerbations cannot be recommended without a multi-faceted self-management programme or ongoing case management.

## Self-management education – individual and group programmes

A particular focus of governmental policy is encouraging patients to become 'experts' in managing their own conditions. A number of systematic reviews have examined the effectiveness of group and individual educational programmes in relation to different LTCs. Van Dam et al.'s (2003) systematic review focused on reviewing studies that educated and empowered patients to participate in care (relating to diabetes) in addition, or in comparison, to altering health care provider behaviour. They concluded that supporting patients to participate in care and self behaviour (through interventions such as assistant-guided patient preparation for visits to doctors, empowering group education, group consultations) was more effective in engaging patients with diabetes in self-care management and positively effecting self-care outcomes, than focusing on their physiological function and modify advice in response to patients in accordance with their bodily cues and experiences (Rees and Williams 2008).

## Who's suitable for self-care?

Numerous reviews and research studies have attempted to determine which patients/clients may be better able to self-manage. When assessing patients it is important that all the factors influencing their current state of health are taken into account and that a holistic approach is taken to care, including reviewing physical, psychological and social need. Some of the potential factors that may influence an individual's ability to self-care have been indicated earlier such as age, disease severity and social support, but it is important to remember that health and social needs change over time. This is particularly relevant for those with LTCs and patients should continue to be provided with the opportunity to self-manage throughout their lifetime. Individuals who prefer their care to be health professional led should not be disadvantaged and should continue to receive the same high standard level of care as those who choose to take a more interactive role. The Flinders Program identify seven characteristics of a 'good' self manager, known as the seven Principles of Self-Management, which refer to the capacity of the individual to:

1. Have knowledge of their condition
2. Follow a treatment plan (care plan) agreed with their health professionals
3. Actively share in decision-making with health professionals
4. Monitor and manage signs and symptoms of their condition
5. Manage the impact of the condition on their physical, emotional and social life
6. Adopt lifestyles that promote health
7. Have confidence, access and the ability to use support services.

(Flinders University 2014)

## Developing concordance/empowerment/shared decision-making/patient-centred care

Issues surrounding behaviour change strategies will be discussed in the next chapter but it is important at this stage to note some of the key terms used when developing the nurse/client relationship to move away from the traditional paradigm of reliance on health care providers and move towards a self-care/self-management paradigm. Shared decision-making is a term very much on today's agenda, not only in relation to LTCs but also with those presenting with more acute self-limiting illnesses. Suffice to say that patient- or person-centred care should involve provision of systems that are patient- rather than service-led, involve individuals with making decisions about their ongoing health care choices, respect those decisions, provide effective treatment, emotional support and empathy, involve families and carers and ensure continuity of care wherever possible. Concordance, rather than compliance, should be the key to all patient/provider interactions, informing individuals about the most effective treatment options and ensuring they understand all the options available, including the pros and cons of choosing or rejecting a plan of care, but respecting their decisions as to how they interpret and apply those treatment options.

## Self-management programmes

### The Chronic Disease Self-Management Programme

Stanford University's Chronic Disease Self-Management Programme developed by Kate Lorig (see Lorig et al. 1999) began initially in the 1970s at the Stanford Patient Education Research Centre, California, USA, originally focusing on self-help skills for people living with arthritis. The theoretical underpinning of the concept is 'self-efficacy', which was developed as a concept by Albert Bandura, a Canadian psychologist, also based at Stanford. The initial Arthritis Self-Help Course, which is now offered world-wide, became the model for a number of other programmes such as the Chronic Disease Self-Management Programme, the Positive Self-Management Programme for HIV/AIDS and the Back Pain Self-Management Programme to name but a few.

The Centre develops and delivers community-based self-management programmes to improve the physical and emotional health of participants living with chronic illness while reducing health care costs, with their main mission being research. All the programmes offered by the centre undergo a rigorous 2–4-year evaluation before being released for wider dissemination. A number of Internet versions of the programmes are currently under evaluation, further details of these can be found at: http://patienteducation. stanford.edu/programs/.

The Chronic Disease Self-Management Programme covers the following key areas:

1. Techniques to deal with problems such as frustration, fatigue, pain and isolation
2. Appropriate exercise for maintaining and improving strength, flexibility, and endurance
3. Appropriate use of medications
4. Communicating effectively with family, friends, and health professionals
5. Nutrition
6. How to evaluate new treatments.

(Stanford University School of Medicine Patient
Education Research Centre 2008)

The Chronic Disease Self-Management Programme has three distinct features: it was developed using the experiences of people living with LTCs as a starting point; is run in community settings and is lay-led by pairs of trained leaders who themselves have an LTC. The programme has since been adopted worldwide (as the EPP in the UK, the Chronic Disease Self-Management Programme in British Columbia, Canada and other adaptations in Europe, Asia, Australia and New Zealand), the key to its success being the way in which it is taught: highly participative classes which encourage mutual support and success to build the participants' confidence in their ability to manage their health and maintain active and fulfilling lives. Programmes are run as interactive workshops over a period of time (generally two hours a week over a six week period), where people with different chronic diseases attend together. It teaches the skills needed in the day-to-day management of treatment and to maintain and/or increase life's activities.

## The Expert Patients Programme (EPP) (UK)

In the UK The Living with Long-term Illness (LILL) Project was set up in September 1998 to increase knowledge about, and the use of, self-management programmes for people living with LTCs. The overall aims included the creation of a self-management information-sharing network, the facilitation of robust monitoring and evaluation processes and the mapping of existing self-management interventions.

The report from this programme fed into the Expert Patients Task Force, set up in 1999 to design a programme that would bring together the valuable work of patient and clinical organisations in developing self-management initiatives. The DH (2001) followed this up with a report *The Expert Patient: A New Approach to Chronic Disease Management for the 21st Century*, which was to lay the foundations for the EPP. Since then the programme, a lay-led self-management programme specifically for people living with LTCs, has grown from strength to strength. In England the EPP currently offers around 12,000 course places a year. Evaluation of the programme indicated that self-management can lead to decreased severity of symptoms and decrease in pain, as well as overall improved life satisfaction and feeling of control, accompanied by increased activity levels. Full details of the evaluation can be obtained from the archived site of the National Primary Care Research & Development Centre: www.population-health.manchester.ac.uk/primarycare/npcrdc-archive/archive/ProjectDetail.cfm/ID/117.htm.

As well as the initial EPP a number of other courses have been developed for groups and communities considered marginalised. These include ethnic minority communities, with courses available in a variety of different languages and courses specifically aimed at groups such as young people living with LTCs, as well as programmes designed for carers.

The EPP has also been rolled out across Wales as EPP Cymru, where it began in 2002. Each session looks at:

- Managing symptoms such as pain and tiredness
- Dealing with anger, fear and frustration
- Coping with stress, depression and low self-image
- Eating healthily
- Learning relaxation techniques and taking regular exercise

- Improving communication with family, friends and health professionals
- Planning for the future.

In addition to the orginal Chronic Disease Self-Management Programme a number of other courses are now also available including Looking After Me (a course for carers) (EPP Cymru 2014).

The overall aim of EPP Cymru is not to review specific individual health needs or provide health condition or treatment information but to encourage people living with LTCs to share their skills and experience and develop the confidence to take responsibility for their own care and to work in equal partnership with health and social care professionals

## Other educational programmes

Although the EPP is the most well known programme and many others have evolved from the initial Chronic Disease Self-Management Programme it is worth noting that there are many other programmes, often specific to particular conditions, that aim to provide individuals with the knowledge and skills with which to manage their own conditions. These include: DAFNE (Dose Adjustment for Normal Eating), DESMOND (Diabetes Education and Self Management for Ongoing and Newly Diagnosed Diabetes), Challenge Arthritis, Self Management for Irritable Bowel Syndrome to name but a few. It is worthwhile determining what is available in your area.

## Key points

- The medical model of care is no longer a suitable model for those with long-term conditions.
- Self-care programmes have been in existence since the 1970s and have been subject to rigorous evaluation studies, although they are not without their critics.
- Inclusion of patient orientated interventions has a far greater impact on health outcomes than concentrating solely on changing provider interventions.
- Not all patients/clients are suitable for self-care, all should be given the opportunity to become involved in self-management but those who choose not to should not be disadvantaged.

## Further areas to consider

- What is the governmental policy regarding delivery of self-care programmes in your area?

- What programmes are available in your area regarding management of chronic illness/LTCs?
- What evaluations are taking place in regards to self-management programmes?
- What systems have been put in place in your practice area to ensure patients are provided with information relating to self-care/self-management?

## Organisations that advise on self-management

A number of charitable organisations provide help and advice to support those suffering with LTCs and some UK examples of these are provided below with the website addresses.

### Arthritis Care

Arthritis Care – *Ways to Self-Manage* (Box 4.4): see www.arthritiscare.org.uk/Living withArthritis/Self-management/Waystoself-manage.

---

### Box 4.4   Ways to self-manage

Self-management is about using your own resources to help manage the condition. There is much you can do for yourself. Indeed, you may well already use a combination of the following techniques:

- keeping active will help keep your muscles strong and joints moving
- looking after your joints by reducing the stress on them
- pacing yourself – try to balance rest with activity
- having a warm bath and using heated pads or a hot water bottle to reduce stiffness
- using a cold pack or a damp cloth around ice cubes or frozen vegetables to reduce swelling
- complementary therapies such as homeopathy, acupuncture and osteopathy
- massage to help relax muscles and improve blood flow
- Tens (Transcutaneous Electrical Nerve Stimulation) machines use electrical impulses to block pain
- relaxation, breathing exercises and meditation techniques to relax muscles and ease pain.

(Arthritis Care 2008)

## Diabetes UK

Diabetes UK – *Managing Your Diabetes* (Box 4.5): see www.diabetes.org.uk/Guide-to-diabetes/Managing-your-diabetes/.

---

### Box 4.5   Taking control of your diabetes

- Get the information you need. The more you know, the more confident you will become and the easier it will be to manage your diabetes.
- Recognise your role: take some personal responsibility for managing your diabetes day-to-day.
- Be honest: give accurate information about your health and how you are really feeling.
- Set goals: put into everyday practice the goals you may have agreed in your care plan.
- Examine your feet regularly between reviews, or ask someone you know to check them for you.
- Ask for help if you are ill, and know the 'sick day rules'.
- Know when, where and how to contact your diabetes health care team.
- Attend your appointments or rearrange them as soon as possible.
- Make a list of points to bring up at your appointments.
- Carry some form of medical identification about your diabetes.
- Discuss with your diabetes health care team if you are pregnant or planning to become pregnant, so that pre- and post-pregnancy advice can be organised with your obstetric team.
- Give feedback to your health care team about the treatment and care you have received.
- Treat NHS staff with respect.

(Diabetes UK 2014)

---

## Asthma UK

Asthma UK – *Living with Asthma* (Box 4.6): see www.asthma.org.uk/knowledge-bank-living-with-asthma.

---

### Box 4.6   Living with asthma

Asthma UK provide a range of publication and advice related to:

- Written asthma action plans
- Travel
- Financial help
- Flu and asthma

other aspects of his identity that do not relate to drinking four pints of beer at the pub quiz may help him to increase his motivation to change this.

## Whether you believe you will be successful

Closely related to how you see yourself is the degree you believe you will be successful in achieving health behaviour changes. This is described within psychological disciplines as self-efficacy (Bandura 1977). It is the single factor that has consistently demonstrated the greatest influence upon outcomes, with higher levels of self-efficacy generally leading to health behaviour changes being made and maintained over time (Conner and Norman 2005). If a person believes they can successfully make a change this is often half the battle. If they do not believe they can change, it may discourage them so much that they may not even want to try (Bandura 1995). Hence, it is really important for health professionals to pay attention to the self-efficacy of the patient to make changes, and support them in building this if it is low.

Thinking again about our patient, Mr Green, if he can imagine succeeding with one small change, this might also help him feel more motivated to work towards it (and maybe others). In clinical situations, practitioners often focus on what the patient has not managed to change. By shifting focus, and concentrating on the small achievements Mr Green has made, this may help him to begin to increase his self-efficacy, which could help him to feel more able to change.

## Inner conflict

When it comes to making changes, reflecting on behaviours that do not match up with our own personal beliefs can also affect our motivation to make changes. Festinger (1957) claimed that a sense of inner conflict ('*cognitive dissonance*') occurs when a person behaves in a certain way, which conflicts with their own beliefs about their self. People generally feel uncomfortable when they hold two conflicting thoughts, and this creates an urge to resolve the conflict.

For example, Mr Green may be thinking 'I want to be healthy, but I eat a lot of food with a lot of fat and sugar in, which is bad for me and my diabetes'. The urge to resolve this conflict could mean that he decides to gradually reduce the amount of saturated fat and sugar in his diet. However, if Mr Green does not believe he can reduce the amount of fat and sugar in his diet very easily, it may be easier to despise what he feels he cannot achieve: 'Who wants to be healthy but unhappy? Let's forget that idea.'

## Ambivalence

In relation to behaviour change, the term 'ambivalence' refers to the notion of having mixed feelings, and in turn feeling unsure or indecisive. Most of us can think of a time in our lives when we have had to make a decision, and have been torn between different courses of action. This may have raised feelings of conflict about which course of action is the best, or a sense of hopelessness when neither path seems to lead to a completely satisfactory ending.

Looking at the example of Mr Green again, we can all see the 'damage' he is doing to his self through eating unhealthy foods, not taking enough exercise and drinking a bit too much alcohol. It is natural to want to stop Mr Green from taking part in these harmful activities – after all, it is often the desire to help and improve the health of others that draws people into careers in health care in the first place.

Mr Green may feel several different ways about making those changes. He can see how changing will be beneficial to his health and quality of life. Conversely however, he may also see that it will be hard to change. Such changes may affect other family members, and he may perceive a negative impact on their social life. He may not enjoy some of the things he has been told he should do, or feel unhappy about giving up behaviours that until now have been pleasurable. This is the essence of ambivalence about making changes to health behaviours, which often makes the decision to change a difficult one.

## Readiness, importance and confidence

Another factor that may affect patient motivation to change is their 'readiness' to make changes. One model commonly used to try to understand readiness is the 'stages of change' component of the transtheoretical model of change (Prochaska and DiClemente 1983). This model describes five possible stages that individuals may be at in terms of making a change:

- Precontemplation stage – the person has not even considered that they might need to make changes at this point
- Contemplation stage – the person has considered that there is something that they probably need to change
- Preparation stage – the person makes plans as to how they might change
- Action stage – the person is actively undertaking behavioural changes
- Maintenance stage – the person maintains the changes they made in the action stage over a period of time.

The stages are not linear – an individual can relapse and fall back into former stages at any point in time. For example, maybe the changes made in the action stage were difficult to implement, causing a person to fall back into the contemplation or preparation stage, or a stressful life event such as a relationship break-up forced the person back into the precontemplation stage for a time.

Two factors that can influence an individual's readiness to make changes are the degree of *importance* they attach to making the behaviour change, and their *confidence* to achieve it (Rollnick et al. 2007; Keller and White 1997). Having the confidence to achieve change is recognised as a great factor in making lifestyle changes. In general, if importance and confidence are both high, the person is more likely to feel ready to make changes. If importance and confidence are both low, they are not likely to feel at all ready to make changes. If importance and confidence are somewhere in the middle of high and low, or either importance or confidence is high but the other is low, the individual is likely to be *ambivalent* about making changes.

Bearing this in mind, if the practitioner could find out where Mr Green is in terms of his readiness to make changes, they can choose the most helpful style in which to talk with him about change. For example, if a practitioner speaks to a patient like they are in the action stage, when in fact they are still contemplating a change, this may lead to the patient actively or passively disengaging with the conversation.

## Health behaviour change interventions

There are a number of health behaviour change interventions employed within primary care settings that have demonstrated effective outcomes. The frameworks provide detail on two broad elements: the 'what' (the content covered) and those with an emphasis on the 'how' (the interactional process).

Current National Institute for Health and Care Excellence (NICE) guidelines on individual behaviour change interventions (NICE 2014d), and the 5 As model for behavioural change counselling (Glasgow et al. 2006; Goldstein et al. 2004) place great emphasis on the 'what' to include in effective behaviour change interventions, but provide relatively little detail on how to actually put this into practice with a patient. However, other interventions such as patient-centred self-management interventions (Roter and Kinmonth 2002), shared decision-making (Makoul and Clayman 2006) and motivational interviewing (Rollnick et al. 2007; Mason and Butler 2010; Miller and Rollnick 2013) place a greater emphasis on relationship building and interaction between practitioners and patients, as this has been shown to be one of the best predictors of behaviour change outcomes (Michael et al. 2012; Hahn 2009; Martin et al. 2005; Najavits et al. 2000). The common content and relational factors that seem to be important in effective health behaviour change interventions are summarised in Table 5.1.

### Pause for reflection

How many documents and guides about health behaviour change skills have you read where there is a heavy emphasis on content? Why might this be? Are there any factors that make focusing on building a good therapeutic relationship with patients within consultations feel more difficult than doing an activity? How could some of these be overcome, despite the barriers?

Summarising the research into what makes an effective health behaviour change intervention in this format should not give the impression that content is superior to relational factors, or vice versa. Nor should it give the impression that there is an

**Table 5.1 Common features that seem to be important in effective health behaviour change interventions**

| *Content* | *Relational factors* |
| --- | --- |
| • Eliciting the patient's understanding around their current health conditions and health behaviours.<br>• Eliciting the patient's past experience of trying to make changes.<br>• Eliciting the patient's understanding of the short-, medium- and long-term consequences of change versus no change.<br>• Providing information to patients that is specifically tailored to their needs and understanding.<br>• Helping the patient to explore the barriers that have prevented change so far, and work out ways to overcome them.<br>• Keeping planned changes small, specific and achievable within a realistic time frame.<br>• Helping the patient to develop an action plan (written down if possible) with specific goals, self-monitoring and regular review.<br>• Helping the patient to developing problem-solving skills and coping strategies, to help plan for difficulties in making changes and relapses.<br>• Helping the patient to identify available social support for making changes.<br>• Planning to have follow-up sessions with the patient to provide support and monitor progress. | • Create a good rapport between you and the patient before engaging in discussions about behaviour change.<br>• Hear and understand the patient's perspective.<br>• Express understanding in a non-judgemental way.<br>• Actively involve the patient in understanding information provided to them, by exploring what they already know, and checking what they have understood.<br>• Treat the patient as the expert in knowing what the best option is for them, and what changes are workable.<br>• Offer choice, and respect patient autonomy in making decisions.<br>• Set goals and create plans etc. in a collaborative manner, drawing upon patient expertise and encouraging them to lead the process.<br>• Focus on what the patient has managed to achieve and highlight this, even when things have not gone exactly to plan.<br>• Offer emotional support if it is needed. |

artificial separation between these two aspects of successfully assisting patients to change their behaviour. Both are fundamental to helping patients to make changes. As 1980s pop group Bananarama explained, quite often, it is not just what we do but the way that we do it that gets results!

For this reason, we shall now spend some time considering the 'how', and the importance skilful communication plays in this, employing a heading inspired by yet another 1980s band.

# Style council

As human beings, we use different styles of communication in different situations within our everyday lives. The styles that we adopt in clinical practice with patients vary – both from patient to patient, and also from issue to issue. We may, for example, find the need to switch styles multiple times during a consultation.

Rollnick et al. (2007) developed a simple three-styles model for understanding how practitioners approach problem solving in everyday practice:

* Directing
* Following
* Guiding.

A *directing* style is widely used in health and social care to solve problems. It involves provision of expert advice and help and done skilfully, is well timed and personally relevant, while not damaging rapport with the patient.

A *following* style describes the approach whereby a clinician offers support and encouragement through careful listening to the patient's situation. The following style is most prevalent in scenarios such as breaking bad news, or when trying to understand why a patient is upset or distressed.

Finally, a *guiding* style involves the clinician and the patient working collaboratively to help the patient identify solutions to a problem. Both the practitioner and patient are active in this process. Guiding can be most effective in discussions about issues such as skill acquisition or making difficult lifestyle changes.

## Pause for reflection

What might the consequences of only using one style of communication in clinical practice be? After looking at theories of behaviour change, why do you think that the guiding style might be better with ambivalent patients, than directing or following?

Skilful communication in practice involves flexibly switching between these styles according to the patient's needs. When it comes to talking about health behaviour changes with ambivalent patients, the guiding style is likely to be most effective.

So, what might guiding actually look like in clinical practice? To illustrate this, we shall now look in more depth at one specific intervention, motivational interviewing (MI). This is because MI has been described as a 'refined form of guiding' (Rollnick et al. 2007), and provides a good example of how to achieve a good therapeutic relationship around behaviour change through using skilful communication. MI is a widely used intervention within health care settings, with good evidence in terms of outcomes. Additionally, MI is a good intervention to use with patients who perhaps feel less ready to change, which makes it a good fit for this chapter.

## Motivational interviewing (MI)

MI is an evidence-based intervention that is used widely by practitioners in the addictions field and beyond. MI has most recently been defined as a 'collaborative, goal-oriented style of communication with particular attention to the language of change . . . designed to strengthen personal motivation and commitment to a specific goal by eliciting and exploring the person's own reasons for change, within an atmosphere of acceptance and compassion' (Miller and Rollnick 2013, p.29). It was originally practised within the addictions field and other specialist, help-seeking clinical settings, with consultation times ranging from approximately thirty minutes to an hour in length. In recent times however, MI has been adapted for use in much briefer consultations in a range of other environments, including general practice settings (Mason and Butler 2010; Rollnick et al. 2007). There is good evidence that MI is an effective health behaviour change intervention within these kinds of settings (Lundahl et al. 2013; Rubak et al. 2005).

As we have seen above, ambivalence can be a barrier to making health behaviour changes. In turn, Miller and Rollnick (2013) argue therefore that resolving ambivalence can in turn be a 'key to change'. Instead of approaching the patient as an individual who does not want to change, by using MI the practitioner focuses on trying to elicit what the patient does want, and how they think they might be able to achieve it.

When talking about ambivalence, patients may produce two different kinds of talk reflecting that ambivalence:

- *Sustain talk* – the costs of changing behaviour, or the benefits of not changing
- *Change talk* – the benefits of changing behaviour, or the costs of not changing.

In MI, the practitioner uses a number of skills to encourage the production of patient change talk. This helps the patient increase their motivation to change their behaviour (Amrhein et al. 2003). This does not mean, however, that sustain talk is avoided in MI. Patient autonomy is respected throughout. Therefore, although sustain talk is not purposely elicited by the health professional, it is accepted and responded to in an empathic and non-judgemental way as part of the process of exploring ambivalence to change.

So, how does MI fit into a guiding style of communication? The practitioner can use a number of skills, such as asking open-ended questions, making summaries and the skilful use of reflective listening to both express empathy and to direct the patient in producing change talk, using these to work collaboratively with the patient, who is the ultimate expert in how and why to make changes to their own health behaviour.

One commonly held misconception of MI is that it is a set of techniques that can be inflicted on a patient, without genuine empathy and understanding. This is not the case. MI is a clinical *skill*, rather than a *tool*. To further define the nature of MI in health care settings, Rollnick et al. (2007) describe the *spirit* of MI in health care (or a 'way of being' with a patient) and present four *principles* (or 'conventions guiding practice'). These are discussed in more detail below.

Pause for reflection

See if you can draw some parallels between the spirit and principles of MI described below, and the theories used to understand behaviour change process discussed above. Also think about how these might relate to the 'how' of the health behaviour change consultation, and why they might be important.

## Motivational interviewing spirit

MI spirit is broken down into three components. In practising MI, a practitioner should aim to be:

- Collaborative
- Evocative
- Honouring patient autonomy.

To work collaboratively, the clinician and patient should aim to work together in partnership – for example, the process should perhaps feel like shared decision-making, rather than the practitioner advocating for change and the patient advocating for no change. A consultation should generally feel like a dance between the patient and the practitioner, rather than a wrestling match. We can see in our example of Mr Green that the practitioner is making all the moves, and Mr Green does not seem to be contributing to the dance very much at all. In fact, his reaction suggests that the practitioner may well have stepped on his toes during the process!

In being evocative, the practitioner elicits the patient's goals, thoughts and feelings about behaviour change, rather than providing information as to how and what they should feel about change. Mr Green's clinician appears to have simply given advice as to what to do, rather than trying to understand why Mr Green does not seem to have made any changes.

Honouring patient autonomy involves signifying respect for the patient's autonomy as an individual to make their own decisions. For example, Mr Green may have his own ideas about changes he might make if he is allowed to go about them in the way that he wants to, in his own time. It is also entirely possible that Mr Green does not want to make any changes. Despite the fact that this is not the best option for his well-being, the practitioner has to accept that Mr Green has made that decision. The ultimate decision about change lies with Mr Green, and Mr Green only.

Later in this chapter, we will focus upon strategies that can be used in health behaviour change consultations. However, it is most important to get the spirit (or the 'how' of the consultation) right. As we have discussed previously, without a good therapeutic relationship, the strategies are unlikely to be effective by themselves and vice versa.

## Motivational interviewing principles

Rollnick et al. (2007) have recently adapted the description of MI principles from the original method to health care contexts. They are described by the acronym RULE:

- Resist the righting reflex
- Understand your patient's motivations
- Listen to your patient
- Empower your patient.

## Resisting the righting reflex

The 'righting reflex' refers to our natural urge as human beings to put things right. For example, if we see somebody who is about to accidentally step out into the path of an oncoming car, it is natural to want to pull them back. Bearing in mind our example of Mr Green, it is clear that the clinician is trying to prevent him coming to any further harm associated with his diabetes and health behaviours. By providing information and advice in the face of Mr Green's ambivalence about change, the practitioner is hoping to save him from himself, creating a feeling of wrestling, rather than dancing. By avoiding this righting reflex, the practitioner could instead try to avoid heightening this discord, and help Mr Green move forward, in a sense continuing the dance rather than the wrestling match. The metaphor of 'wrestling' describes a process described as 'discord' (Miller and Rollnick 2013), which indicates that the therapeutic relationship between the patient and the practitioner is breaking down in some way. The practitioner can attempt to restore the therapeutic relationship by perhaps 'going along with what the patient says for a bit' while demonstrating understanding for the patient's reaction as a means of reducing it (for example, by saying something like 'It sounds like you think I'm going to try to force you to do things you're not happy with').

## Understand your patient's motivations

This involves listening carefully to your patient's reasons for and against change. What is it that makes them ambivalent about change? Listen carefully to their sustain talk and their change talk, as this will give you more information about why the patient is where they are at the current time. For example, why does Mr Green's busy life make it more difficult to make health behaviour changes? What kinds of things hold him back? If he was going to make some changes, how might he go about it? The health professional Mr Green saw might have used their time more effectively with regards to facilitating change by asking these kinds of questions, rather than telling him what he should do and how he should do it (which seems not to have been an effective strategy thus far).

# Health behaviour change strategies

In addition to paying attention to the 'how' within the behaviour change consultation, we need to make sure that we do not forget the 'what' or content aspects as part of that process. There are a number of strategies drawn from both the MI and the wider health behaviour change interventions literature discussed above that can be helpful within behaviour change consultations. These can be useful in encouraging the exploration of ambivalence, emphasising personal choice and autonomy, and helping patients feel understood. For more guidance on the skilful use of these strategies, take a look at Mason and Butler (2010).

## Pause for reflection

As you are reading through these strategies, think about how you might be able to integrate these into a patient care plan, and how you might document this. Are there any worksheets or resources you could create to help you and your patients?

# Agenda setting and permission seeking

Given that lack of choice in talking about behaviour change can be one of the things that can increase resistance, it is a good idea to encourage the patient to be active in choosing to talk about behaviour change. After all, talking about behaviour change should ultimately be the patient's choice.

The first thing the practitioner can do to this end is to ask permission to talk about the behaviour with the patient, rather than just telling the patient that today there will be a discussion about their health behaviour. Perhaps saying to Mr Green 'I'm just wondering if it would be alright to have a quick chat with you about your diet in relation to your diabetes. Would that be OK?', rather than simply telling him what to do, might help him feel a little more in control.

Encouraging the patient to suggest what behaviour changes they would like to talk about is particularly important if there are a number of different lifestyle issues to be addressed. For example, Mr Green could benefit from making some changes to his diet, taking a bit more exercise and cutting down on his alcohol intake.

It is often easier to make changes gradually, rather than trying to make a number of substantial changes all in one go. Achieving small changes is a great way to help a patient boost their sense of self-efficacy (Bandura 1977). A patient is more likely to feel more able to make other changes if they have already succeeded with one small change. Starting where the patient feels most comfortable, and encouraging them to suggest what area they would like to talk about, is useful for both helping patients to feel more in control of talking about behaviour change, and for starting where they feel most ready to make changes.

So, how can we encourage the patient to set the agenda? After all, this might be something they are not used to in a consultation.

This can be approached through the use of open questions, such as 'There are a number of different things we can talk about today, Mr Green. What is it that you would like to talk to me about today?'

One clinical tool that can help with this task is an 'agenda setting chart' (Mason and Butler 2010), which contains a number of circles containing picture representations of different lifestyle factors, and some blank circles. The blank circles are for other factors to be inserted by the patient. This means that sometimes the practitioner needs to be prepared for the patient to raise issues that they have not previously expected – for example, perhaps Mr Green is concerned about how the level of stress in his life is currently affecting his diabetes, rather than what he is eating at the moment.

---

## Pause for reflection

How might you go about setting an agenda with your own patients in a guiding style that helps you to build a good therapeutic relationship at the same time?

---

## Exploring how the patient feels about change

As we have seen, how ready the patient feels about change can impact directly on their motivation to make changes, so spending some time exploring those reasons with the patient is important.

One way this can be achieved within clinical practice is by exploring how important the patient feels it is to change their behaviour, and how confident he or she feels in achieving it. Asking 'scaling questions' to do this can be useful. This involves asking the patient on a scale of 0–10 how important is it for them to change a particular behaviour, and then ask on the same scale how confident they feel about successfully making that change. Following on from this, there is the opportunity to ask the patient why they have given themselves this score and not a higher or lower number, or indeed what they think would help them to move up the scale in terms of importance and/or confidence.

Of course, you can do this without asking scaling questions. Importance and confidence could equally be assessed by the use of skilful, open questions, such as 'How important would you say it is for you to make changes to your diet, Mr Green?' and 'If you made the decision that you were going to change what you eat, how confident are you that you would succeed?'

Another way to help the patient explore how they feel about making changes is to help them identify what they like/dislike about their current behaviour, and what they feel they would gain/lose from changing. This is an ideal opportunity for the clinician to elicit change talk from the patient and to reinforce that through reflective listening.

Pause for reflection

How important do you think it is to try and incorporate some of these strategies into your practice, along with MI skills, principles and spirit? How confident are you that you will succeed?

## Exchanging information

Obviously within health care consultations, there are times when patients need information or advice. Perhaps the patient needs to know something for their safety or well-being, they have asked you for information on what they should do, or they have misunderstood something with regards to their care or recovery.

Information giving within health care is usually a process in which the patient is a passive recipient. Using Mr Green as an example, the health care professional might have said something like 'Your HbA1c is still at 10.5. Really, we need to get it down to about 6.5. You need to start taking more care of yourself and eating less convenience foods – get a little more fruit and vegetables into your diet. If you don't, then you are putting yourself at risk of complications. You could go blind! I'm sure you don't want that to happen.' This has the advantage of being direct and to the point. However, on the down side, Mr Green might know all this already, or perhaps he does not see how this is relevant to him. It also makes the assumption that Mr Green will just take the advice and do as he is told. We know this is not the case with ambivalent patients, because Mr Green has been back time and again, and still not implemented any of the advice he has been given.

As we observed from the common factors in effective health behaviour change interventions, it is more helpful to actively *exchange* information with patients, rather than to position them as a passive recipient of the information. One useful strategy for doing this is the *'elicit-provide-elicit'* method. This involves first finding out what the patient knows already, providing further information (with patient permission) and then finding out what the patient has made of that information. An example of this might be:

- Elicit: 'So Mr Green, how much do you know about the complications of diabetes?'
- Provide: 'Would it be OK if I told you a little bit more about that?'
- Elicit: 'So, what do you think that might mean for you and your diabetes?'

Exchanging information in this way can encourage the patient to actively think of how the information given applies to their self as an individual, and it can even save the clinician time, as it prevents the provision of information that the patient already knows about. The information is given in a neutral manner, and builds on the patient's existing knowledge. Leaving the interpretation of the facts to the patient helps them to recognise what the personal relevance of the information is – rather than listening to the reasons why the practitioner thinks this information is relevant.

---

**Pause for reflection**

---

Think about some of the information you are required to give to patients. How might it look in practice if you were to deliver the same information using the elicit-provide-elicit method? What might the advantages be?

---

## Setting goals

If a patient indicates that they are ready to make changes, the most useful course of action is to elicit from the patient what changes they feel they would like to make. By focusing on small changes that feel achievable, this can help the patient feel more confident of success and more able to face other changes (Bandura 1977). If multiple or larger changes need to be made, it may be easier for the patient to break these changes down into smaller tasks, rather than trying to do it all at once.

The health professional who Mr Green saw no doubt has years of experience in clinical practice and knows exactly what he needs to do to achieve better diabetes control. However, as it is Mr Green who has to make these changes, he is the expert, as he knows what will work best for him. The patient should be an active decision-maker, rather than a passive recipient of information and advice.

How might we go about drawing this out of Mr Green? Using some good open questions such as 'What sorts of things do you think you might be able to do?' might be helpful to start things off. This does not mean that the health professional cannot offer possible courses of action to the patient – Mr Green might even ask for advice about what he could do. Before making a suggestion however, it is a good idea to ask permission, and emphasise that it is up to the patient to decide if they think it will be useful for them. For example the clinician might say something like 'Trying to fit exercise into your everyday life, so that you don't have to change your routine too much sounds like it might be the most workable for you. Some of the patients I see say that they try to take a 10-minute walk after their dinner in the evening. Do you think that's something that might work for you, or do you think you might need to try something different?'

Another thing that can be helpful is to encourage the patient to think about previous attempts to change their behaviour. For example, asking Mr Green what has worked well before, what kinds of things did not work, and why, might help him to think about different things that he might try to make changes this time.

When planning changes to be made, it is important to focus on something specific that can be monitored, rather than something vague. Not having a clear idea of exactly what it is that is being worked on in the short term can make it more difficult for a patient to focus once they leave the consultation. The following questions can be helpful for patients who are setting a goal:

- What specifically do you plan to do? (e.g. reduce my alcohol intake)
- What do you think is the first step? (e.g. I am going to try to drink three pints of beer instead of four when I go out)

- How do you think you will go about it? (e.g. on Wednesday when I am at the pub quiz, and in the pub on Saturday and Sunday, I'll drink my beer more slowly and perhaps drink water when I've had three pints)
- How confident do you feel that you can achieve this on a scale from 0–10? (e.g. about a 6, because it seems doable, but I think when I'm in the moment with my friends, it could be a bit tricky)
- How will you know your plan is working? (e.g. when I get into a regular habit of only having three pints so it feels normal, and I've found a comfortable way to manage to say no to my friends when I've had my three).
- How could you monitor this? (e.g. keep a note each time I've been to the pub of the number of pints I've had, how I've dealt with my friends and how well that has worked).

## Pause for reflection

What strategies could you put in place to help you to guard against telling your patients what changes they need to make, and help you to encourage your patient to set their own goals?

## Problem solving and planning for difficulties

Think about times when you have tried to make a change, and what it has been like to try to keep that change going over time. You can guarantee that sometimes, despite how much we want to make a change, and no matter how well planned that change is, we run into difficulties in our daily lives that interfere with our plans.

Often, this can lead to a 'roadblock' – something that is standing in the way of our change and is preventing us moving forward with this. It can be difficult to see a way around a roadblock in the moment, and many people find that this can lead to them giving up on changes and falling back into old habits. This in itself can lead to a reduction in a person's self-efficacy about succeeding with lifestyle changes, which is not good given the importance of self-efficacy in clinical outcomes.

So, what might we be able to do to help Mr Green with this? We can see that Mr Green often leads with the best of intentions, but reports he has been unable to make the changes he planned due to being busy, and feeling tired. This suggests that being busy and tiredness are 'roadblocks' for Mr Green. This is valuable information, as it helps us to anticipate difficulties that may show up, and this gives Mr Green an opportunity to plan for these obstacles. The health professional can help by asking open questions, such as 'You said earlier that being busy sometimes prevented you from eating healthily. What do you think you could do to help you to continue with your plans at times when you are busy?' This gives Mr Green an opportunity to think ahead and make contingency plans for this particular roadblock. Patients sometimes find 'if . . . then' planning helpful in this respect, writing down their contingency plans:

'If (x happens), then I will . . . instead'. This kind of approach would enable Mr Green to have a number of pre-planned alternative routes around this roadblock before he reaches it.

So, then what happens when something Mr Green did not anticipate jumps up and presents itself as a roadblock? Let's say for example, that when Mr Green and his wife go to the supermarket, there are three for two offers on some rather delicious cakes, and rather than having the one slice he planned and freezing the rest, he and Mrs Green ate them all in a weekend.

It is important to prepare patients for these kinds of experiences before they happen. Experiencing lapses like this are completely normal in the process of making and maintaining changes, yet they can often lead to a patient thinking 'Oh well, I've blown it now, what's the point', and falling back into old behaviours, so it is important to highlight this at the outset. For example, the health professional might say something like 'It can be really difficult to maintain changes, and things can pop up in our lives that may knock us off track. This is really normal, and it is really important to remember that it is just one event. It doesn't have to stop us making changes in the long term, even if it's standing in the way in the short term. It's also really helpful when this happens, as we have the opportunity to learn about the things that get in our way so we can plan for them'.

In talking about lapses, it can be helpful to encourage the patient to reflect on the following:

- What led up to the lapse? What situation were you in, how were you feeling, what was going through your mind? (e.g. I'd really enjoyed that piece of cake earlier, my wife was having another piece and I felt I didn't want to go without, I really wanted one too, I knew I shouldn't but I couldn't resist it, then I ate another large piece).
- How did you feel after the lapse? What did you think? What did you do? (e.g. I felt really angry with myself, then I thought 'I've blown it, what's the point of trying to change' and just carried on eating cake throughout the day and the day after).
- If you were confronted with this roadblock again, what would you like to do differently? (e.g. I'd prefer not to buy as much cake next time, as this makes me want to eat more of it when it is in the house. I would like to just draw a line under it when I've eaten more than I planned, rather than getting angry with myself and giving up).
- What do you think you will do now? (e.g. I am going to write an 'if . . . then' plan around eating too much and getting angry at myself. I will ask myself 'do I need it?' when I see three for two offers in the supermarket).

## Social support

There is evidence that having support from others is beneficial in making and maintaining health behaviour changes (Gallant 2014). Encouraging patients to think about their own social networks, in terms of who might be able to help them with their changes and how specifically they might be able to help, can be beneficial to them in terms of managing changes outside the clinical consultation. For patients with limited social networks, exploring ways to help them engage with others and expand their social networks can be highly beneficial in terms of clinical outcomes (Uchino 2006).

## Follow-up

There is evidence to suggest that patients who are offered regular follow-up seem to do better at maintaining changes than those who are not (Fjeldsoe et al. 2011). This may potentially be because this creates a space for patients to reflect on progress, identify difficulties and problem solve as described above (Cavill et al. 2011).

## Developing health behaviour change skills

In this chapter, we have explored the process of behaviour change, and looked at the issue of patients who are ambivalent to change, and what might be helpful. We have looked at the spirit and principles of MI, communication skills and health behaviour change strategies you might want to employ whilst using an MI approach, and the evidence for using MI in practice.

However, this chapter has only touched on the basics of health behaviour change and MI. You might feel that you would like some more detailed description about how you can incorporate this into your practice, and indeed, to have some formal training to develop your skills.

Publications such as Rollnick et al. (2007), Miller and Rollnick (2013), Mason and Butler (2010), Shumaker et al. (2009), Berry (2007) and Martin and DiMatteo (2014), which you can find in the References, describe the processes outlined above in much more detail. You might find reading these publications useful, as well as reviewing the references throughout this chapter.

The Motivational Interviewing Network of Trainers (MINT) advertises courses being run by its members all over the world, and lists MI trainers who are willing to deliver MI training specifically in relation to health behaviour change, on its website: www.motivationalinterview.org. You will also find lots of other helpful resources on this website about learning MI, including instruments to assess clinical skills in MI. After initial MI training, Rosengren (2009) and Schumacher and Madson (2014) are useful manuals to help practitioners continue to develop their skills beyond training workshops.

For readers based in the UK, there are also some free e-learning courses on health behaviour change, communication skills, motivational interviewing and shared decision-making available from www.healthscotland.com, and by clicking on your region at www.hee.nhs.uk.

## Key points

- Many patients are ambivalent about making changes, which can affect their motivation to make changes.
- MI is a refined form of a guiding style of communication that aims to help patients explore and resolve ambivalence to change.
- There are many skills and strategies a practitioner can use in the behaviour change consultation, but it is as important to pay attention to the 'how' as well as the 'what'.
- There are resources you can access to try to help you learn more about health behaviour change, and develop your own skills.
- No matter how much you try, you cannot *make* somebody change!

## Further areas to consider

- How useful do you think these ideas could be to you in clinical practice?
- What can you do next to further develop your skills in health behaviour change?
- To what extent do you think you could integrate MI and health behaviour change strategies into your own clinical practice?
- What are the challenges to implementing MI and health behaviour change strategies in clinical practice? What kinds of things could help you?

<table>
<tr><td>6</td><td></td></tr>
</table>

# How to identify a person with a long-term condition

**6**

---

### Overview

A definition of what a long-term condition (LTC) constitutes and what types of condition can be considered as long term has been supplied in the earlier chapters. This chapter is a practical guide to straightforward diagnostic criteria (where these exist) of some of the conditions that constitute an LTC e.g. diabetes, asthma, chronic obstructive pulmonary disease (COPD) etc. For conditions that have more complex diagnostic criteria such as cardiovascular disease (CVD), epilepsy, arthritis etc., a brief overview is provided with reference to appropriate texts. The aim is not to supply detailed manuals on every LTC but to discuss general principles relating to identification and diagnosis.

---

## Introduction

Previous chapters have discussed the varying types of condition that can be considered to be long term. These range greatly in type, presentation and prevalence. In Chapter 2 the World Health Organisation (WHO) definition of an LTC was used to demonstrate that the term LTC should no longer be confined to conditions of greatest prevalence, or to those that lead to the highest mortality rates, but should include any condition, physical/structural or mental, that impacts on health, will worsen without health care intervention and/or behaviour change on the part of the individual and for which at the present time there is no defined cure.

This chapter will provide diagnostic criteria, where available, relating to some of the LTCs discussed in Chapter 2 to provide the reader with some practical guidance regarding appropriate screening, detection and diagnosis of an LTC. The criteria used are those currently recommended in the UK, and are generally based on the National Institute for Health and Care Excellence (NICE) guidance and NICE Clinical Knowledge Summaries (CKS) which provide primary care practitioners with readily accessible summaries of current evidence and clinical guidance on best practice. NICE commission the National Clinical Guideline Centre (NGCC) to develop clinical practice guidelines and each guideline is overseen by an independent guideline development group (GDG). The NGCC was formed in April 2009 following the merger of the National Collaborating Centres for Acute Care, Chronic Conditions, Nursing and Supportive Care and Primary Care.

Some reference will be made to the differences in other countries, particularly regarding diagnostic criteria, but users who are not UK based should ensure that they consult the correct criteria for their own country and not rely solely on those provided in this book. You should also be aware that diagnostic criteria are subject to regular updating; what is accurate today may be out of date next year. To this end the sources of the criteria will be provided and the reader should ensure they access these sources to support them when making a diagnosis. Where firm diagnostic criteria do not currently exist, the signs and symptoms of the condition will be discussed, although again the reader should be aware that diagnosis is a complex art and appropriate medical professionals should always be involved in discussions relating to individual diagnosis. Although general treatment principles for LTCs have been discussed throughout this book and examples of care using case studies will be provided in Chapter 10, specific treatment for individual conditions is not discussed and readers should refer to appropriate evidence-based guidelines (details in Chapter 9) for more precise treatment procedures.

## Conditions

### Diabetes mellitus

#### Classification of diabetes and disorders of glucose homeostasis

There are five clinical categories of disordered glucose homeostasis:

* Type 1 diabetes
* Type 2 diabetes
* Impaired glucose tolerance/impaired fasting glucose
* Gestational diabetes
* Other specific types: including a number of endocrine, infectious and rare genetic conditions affecting the exocrine pancreas, drug and chemical related causes and the genetic condition maturity-onset diabetes in the young (MODY).

(British Medical Association (BMA) 2004)

The following signs and symptoms should alert health care professionals to the possibility of diabetes:

* Weight loss
* Polydipsia (excessive thirst)
* Polyuria (increased urine production)
* Incontinence

- Tiredness/lethargy
- Recurrent infections e.g. thrush, cystitis, balanitis
- Mood changes
- Altered vision
- Foot ulceration
- Delayed wound healing
- Ketoacidosis.

NICE is currently developing four new pieces of guidance relating to diabetes with an anticipated publication date of August 2015: Diabetes in children (Types 1 and 2), Diabetes in pregnancy, Type 1 diabetes in adults, Type 2 diabetes in adults.

## Differentiation between types

TYPE 1 DIABETES

Type 1 diabetes is classically a disease of the young but can occur at any age, onset is generally rapid and presentation acute. Type 1 diabetes clusters in families, about 10 per cent of people diagnosed have a first degree relative with the condition (CKS 2010a). Causation in the majority of cases is an auto-immune process which destroys the insulin producing pancreatic beta cells. Both genetic and environmental factors have been implicated as important factors in the initiation of this process, with a growing body of evidence suggesting that unknown infectious agents or components of early childhood diet can trigger the development of auto-immunity to the beta cells in the Islets of Langerhans in the pancreas (CKS 2010a). The process of pancreatic beta cell destruction normally takes place over a few weeks with symptoms becoming apparent as glucose levels build up due to the lack of insulin. Type 1 diabetes should be suspected in a patient of any age who presents with sudden weight loss and raised blood glucose. The presence of ketonuria in the absence of fasting can aid in the differentiation between type 1 and type 2 diabetes (BMA 2004).

In adults with suspected type 1 diabetes where classical symptoms are present diagnosis can be confirmed by a single laboratory glucose measurement; this should be repeated if classical symptoms are not present (NICE 2004). A full medical, environmental, cultural and educational assessment should be performed to develop an individualised and culturally appropriate care plan, including choice of insulin and insulin regime, self-monitoring of blood glucose and education relating to dietary management and lifestyle (NICE 2004). This should be negotiated between the professional team and the person with type 1 diabetes and implemented without inappropriate delay (NICE 2004). Without treatment diabetic ketoacidosis (DKA) (see Chapter 2) can develop which can lead to coma and eventually death. Additional symptoms that indicate DKA include:

- vomiting
- stomach pain
- rapid breathing
- increased pulse rate
- sleepiness.

TYPE 2 DIABETES

Type 2 diabetes is generally preceded by an asymptomatic period of impaired glucose tolerance, which is characterised by a response to an oral glucose challenge that is not normal, but is not diagnostic of diabetes (BMA 2004). Type 2 diabetes is the most common type of diabetes, accounting for 90–95 per cent of all cases of diabetes with prevalence increasing with age; it is frequently undiagnosed with many people being unaware of their condition (NICE 2009b; CKS 2010b). Particular conditions can increase the risk of type 2 diabetes including: cardiovascular disease, hypertension, obesity, stroke, polycystic ovary syndrome, a history of gestational diabetes and mental health problems. People with learning disabilities and those attending accident and emergency, emergency medical admissions units, vascular and renal surgery units and ophthalmology departments may also be at high risk (NICE 2012b). Although type 2 diabetes has characteristically been thought of as a condition affecting the middle aged and elderly, type 2 diabetes is increasingly been detected in younger people, including children. People are normally thought to have type 2 diabetes if they do not have type 1 diabetes (rapid onset, often in childhood, insulin-dependent, ketoacidosis if neglected) or other medical conditions or treatment suggestive of secondary diabetes. Type 1 diabetes should be considered if ketonuria is detected or if weight loss is marked (NICE 2004).

The distinction between type 1 and type 2 diabetes can however be blurred, with some patients presenting with type 2 having an incomplete form of type 1 disease. There can also be uncertainty in the diagnosis in overweight people of younger age (National Collaborating Centre for Chronic Conditions (NCC-CC) 2008). The possibility of type 2 diabetes should be suspected in younger people presenting with symptoms of diabetes who are obese, have a family history of type 2 diabetes or are of non-white ethnicity (NICE 2004). The risk factors relating to development of type 2 diabetes include obesity, particularly central abdominal obesity, reduced physical activity and genetic predisposition (including ethnicity), as well as intrauterine factors. Insulin resistance, initial hyperinsulinaemia and later beta cell destruction resulting in reduced insulin levels are well recognised in the pathogenesis of type 2 diabetes (BMA 2004).

The WHO recommendations for definition and diagnosis of diabetes mellitus and intermediate hyperglycaemia were reviewed in 2006. The issues discussed included whether the current diabetes diagnostic criteria should be changed, how should normal plasma glucose levels, impaired glucose tolerance and impaired fasting glucose be defined and what tests should be used to define glycaemic status. Based on data available at the time and current recommendations a number of recommendations were made and these are summarised below:

- Current WHO diagnostic criteria of fasting plasma glucose (FPG) $\geq 7.0$mmol/l (126mg/dl) **or** 2–h plasma glucose $\geq 11.1$mmol/l (200mg/dl) should be maintained as these criteria identify a group with significantly increased premature mortality and increased risk of microvascular and cardiovascular complications.
- 'Normoglycaemia' should be used for glucose levels associated with low risk of developing diabetes or cardiovascular disease.
- The current WHO recommendation for Impaired Glucose Tolerance (IGT) should remain at present; consideration should be given to replacing this by an overall

risk assessment for diabetes and CVD, including a measure of glucose as a continuous variable.

- The fasting plasma glucose cut-point for Impaired Fasting Glucose (IFG) should remain at 6.1mmol/l; consideration should be given to replacing this by an overall risk assessment for diabetes and CVD, including a measure of glucose as a continuous variable.
- Venous plasma glucose should be the standard method for measuring and reporting glucose concentrations in blood, although as many under-resourced countries use capillary sampling, conversion values for post load glucose values are provided within the document, fasting values are identical.
- The oral glucose tolerance test (OGTT) should be retained as a diagnostic test as FPG fails to identify 30 per cent of undiagnosed cases, OGTT is the only means of identifying people with IGT, OGTT is often require to exclude or confirm abnormal glucose tolerance in asymptomatic people. An OGTT should be used in individuals with fasting plasma glucose 6.1–6.9mmol/l (110–125mg/dl) to determine glucose tolerance status.

(WHO 2006b)

In 2011 the WHO recommended that glycated haemoglobin (HbA1c) could be used as an alternative to standard glucose measures to diagnose type 2 diabetes among non-pregnant adults. HbA1c levels of 48 mmol/mol (6.5 per cent) or above indicate that someone has type 2 diabetes. However, the WHO did not provide specific guidance on HbA1c criteria for people at increased risk of type 2 diabetes (WHO 2011). The NICE (2012b) guideline *Preventing Type 2 Diabetes: Risk Identification and Interventions for Individuals at High Risk* further notes that a report from a UK expert group recommends using HbA1c values between 42 and 47 mmol/mol (6.0–6.4 per cent) to indicate that a person is at high risk of type 2 diabetes. The group also recognised that there is a continuum of risk across a range of sub-diabetic HbA1c levels – and that people with an HbA1c below 42 mmol/mol (6.0 per cent) may also be at risk. The NICE guideline includes a flowchart for identifying and managing people at moderate and high risk of developing diabetes and those with possible type 2 diabetes.

Box 6.1 summarises the WHO (2006b; 2011) recommendations.

---

## Box 6.1   WHO recommendations for definition and diagnosis of diabetes mellitus and intermediate hyperglycaemia

### Diabetes mellitus

Fasting plasma glucose ≥7.0mmol/l (126mg/dl)
or
2–h plasma glucose* ≥11.1mmol/l (200mg/dl)

*(continued)*

*(continued)*

## Impaired Glucose Tolerance (IGT)

Fasting plasma glucose <7.0mmol/l (126mg/dl)
and
2–h plasma glucose* ≥7.8 and <11.1mmol/l
(140mg/dl and 200mg/dl)

## Impaired Fasting Glucose (IFG)

Fasting plasma glucose 6.1 to 6.9mmol/l
(110mg/dl to 125mg/dl)
and (if measured)
2–h plasma glucose* <7.8mmol/l (140mg/dl)

---

* Venous plasma glucose 2 hours after ingestion of 75g oral glucose load
* If 2-hour plasma glucose is not measured, status is uncertain as diabetes or IGT cannot be excluded

(WHO 2006b, p.3)

**HbA1c** can be used as a diagnostic test for diabetes providing that stringent quality assurance tests are in place and assays are standardised to criteria aligned to the international reference values, and there are no conditions present which preclude its accurate measurement.

An HbA1c of 48 mmol/mol (6.5 per cent) is recommended as the cut point for diagnosing diabetes. A value of less than 48 mmol/mol does not exclude diabetes diagnosed using glucose tests (WHO 2011).

Diagnosis of diabetes requires careful substantiation with retesting on another day unless the person is symptomatic and the plasma glucose is unequivocally elevated.

Although both the American Diabetic Association (ADA) and the previous 1999 WHO criteria for diagnosing diabetes previously defined normal plasma glucose levels, the current WHO criteria recommends that since there are insufficient data to accurately define normal glucose levels, the term 'normoglycaemia' should be used for glucose levels associated with low risk of developing diabetes or CVD, that is levels below those used to define intermediate hyperglycaemia.

Following confirmation of diagnosis a full clinical assessment should be performed prior to an agreed treatment plan being initiated. This should include full medical examination, body mass index and waist measurement, blood pressure, cardiovascular risk assessment, referral for retinal photography, foot examination including

interpreting readings, as vessels are likely to be incompressible and results artificially high. Young and otherwise healthy adults, presenting prematurely with claudication, should be referred to exclude entrapment syndromes and other rare disorders.

## Chronic kidney disease (CKD)

The NICE (2014c) clinical guideline *Chronic Kidney Disease: Early Identification and Management of Chronic Kidney Disease in Adults in Primary and Secondary Care* provides new and updated areas including identification and investigation of people at risk of developing CKD, classification of CKD, definition of CKD progression as well as self-management and pharmacotherapy. NICE (2014c) recommend testing for CKD using eGFR and albumin:creatinine ratio should be offered once a year to people with the following risk factors: diabetes; hypertension; acute kidney injury; CVD; structured renal tract disease; multisystem disease with potential kidney involvement; family history of end stage or hereditary kidney disease; opportunistic detection of haematuria and in people prescribed known nephrotoxic drugs. People should be advised not to eat meat in the 12 hours before having a blood test for eGFR, blood samples should be processed by the laboratory within 12 hours of venepuncture. An ethnicity correction value should be applied for people of African-Caribbean ethnicity, correct identification and assessment of older people requires added caution, as do results in people with extremes of muscle mass.

CKD is defined according to the presence or absence of kidney damage and level of kidney function – irrespective of the type of kidney disease. The classification of CKD has evolved over time; it was initially based on the American National Kidney Foundation Kidney Disease Outcomes Quality Initiative (NKF KDOQI) guidelines (Renal Association 2007; see Renal Association 2013 for 2013 guidelines). Two key changes were suggested to this classification by NICE in 2008 to delineate an increased risk of adverse outcomes; further categories were included in 2013 and are shown in Table 6.1.

People with CKD should be offered education and information tailored to the severity and cause, associated complications and risk of progression. Renal ultrasound should be offered to those with accelerated progression; visible or persistent invisible haematuria, symptoms of urinary tract obstruction; family history of polycystic kidney disease, GFR of less than 30ml/min/1.73m² or those considered by a nephrologist to require a renal biopsy.

## Epilepsy

Epilepsy is a difficult condition to diagnose; with misdiagnosis common, it is recommended that all adults having a first seizure and children having a first non-febrile seizure should be seen within 14 days of referral by a specialist medical practitioner or paediatrician with training and expertise in epilepsy (CKS 2014b;

Table 6.1 Classification of chronic kidney disease using GFR and ACR categories

| GFR and ACR categories and risk of adverse outcomes | | | ACR categories (mg/mmol), description and range | | | |
|---|---|---|---|---|---|---|
| | | | <3 Normal to mildly increased | 3–30 Moderately increased | >30 Severely increased | |
| | | | A1 | A2 | A3 | |
| GFR categories (ml/min/1.73m²), description and range | ≥90 Normal and high | G1 | No CKD in the absence of markers of kidney damage | | | Increasing risk |
| | 60–89 Mild reduction related to normal range for a young adult | G2 | | | | |
| | 45–59 Mild–moderate reduction | G3a[1] | | | | |
| | 30–44 Moderate–severe reduction | G3b | | | | |
| | 15–29 Severe reduction | G4 | | | | |
| | <15 Kidney failure | G5 | | | | |

Increasing risk →

[1] Consider using eGFRcystatinC for people with CKD G3aA1 (see recommendations 1.1.14 and 1.1.15)

Abbreviations: ACR, albumin:creatinine ratio; CKD, chronic kidney disease; GFR, glomerular filtration rate

Adapted with permission from Kidney Disease: Improving Global Outcomes (KDIGO) CKD Work Group (2013) KDIGO 2012 clinical practice guideline for the evaluation and management of chronic kidney disease. *Kidney International* (Suppl. 3): 1–150

NICE 2012c). This will ensure precise and early diagnosis and treatment initiation appropriate to need. Within primary care it is recommended that where seizure is suspected a detailed description should be obtained about the seizure, preferably from a first-hand witness (if available). People with suspected epilepsy should be advised to stop driving, avoid swimming and bathe under supervision. Written information should be provided about what happens during an epileptic seizure and what to expect when they see the specialist. They should be asked to take a witness of the seizure to their first hospital appointment if possible and contact the GP if further episodes occur whilst they are waiting to see a specialist; the GP should seek specialist advice if concerned about recurrent episodes (CKS 2014b; NICE 2012c).

Specialist diagnosis will include detailed history of the attack and symptoms from the person who experienced the attack and eye witness(es). EEG can be used to support diagnosis, neuroimaging may be used to identify structural abnormalities that cause certain epilepsies, MRI is the imaging investigation of choice (NICE 2012b).

## Dementia

Diagnosis of dementia is complex and should only be made after a comprehensive assessment that should include: history taking; cognitive and mental state examination; physical examination and other appropriate investigations; medication review to identify and minimise use of drugs, including over the counter products that may affect cognitive functioning. A number of tools are available to assess cognitive impairment and formal neuropsychological testing should form part of the assessment where dementia is mild or questionable. Assessment should be made at diagnosis and at regular intervals for medical conditions and key psychiatric features associated with dementia (NICE 2012a).

## Respiratory conditions

### Asthma

This section is based on diagnostic criteria in children and adults as detailed in the British Thoracic Society (BTS)/SIGN (2014) guidelines. Although this book mainly concentrates on LTCs in adults, asthma in both adults and children is a common problem seen in the primary care environment and so diagnostic criteria for both are detailed here.

### *Diagnosis in children*

Asthma causes recurrent respiratory systems of wheezing, cough, difficulty breathing and chest tightness in children. Wheezing should be distinguished from stridor or rattly breathing and it is important to be aware that there are many causes of wheezing in childhood. Diagnosis of asthma is based on recognising an episodic pattern of signs and symptoms with no alternative explanation. BTS/SIGN (2014) outline the clinical features that increase the probability of asthma in children as:

- More than one of the following: wheezing, cough, difficulty breathing and chest tightness, particularly if these are frequent or recurrent, worse at night/early in the

morning, occur in response to, or are worse after, triggers such as exercise, pets, cold air, emotions or laughter, or occur after colds
- Personal history of atopic disorder
- Family history of asthma/atopic disorder
- Widespread wheeze detected on chest auscultation
- History of improvement in symptoms or lung function in response to adequate therapy.

A number of factors, outlined in the guidelines, make a diagnosis of asthma more likely, with family atopy, particularly maternal atopy, the most clearly defined risk factor. Assessment of suspected asthma in children should be based on the presence of key features in the history and examination and careful consideration of alternative diagnoses. BTS/SIGN (2014) advise that based on initial clinical assessment it should be possible to determine the probability of a diagnosis of asthma and suggest:

- Children with a high probability of asthma should be put straight onto a trial of treatment with response reviewed and further testing arranged for those with poor response.
- Children with a low probability of asthma should be further investigated and referred for specialist assessment.
- In children with an intermediate probability of asthma who can perform spirometry and have evidence of airways obstruction, change in response to an inhaled bronchodilator and/or response to a trial treatment should be assessed. If there is significant reversibility or if a treatment trial is beneficial treatment should be considered at the minimum effective dose with a trial of reduction or withdrawal of treatment attempted at a later date. If there is evidence of airways obstruction and no significant reversibility and treatment trial is not beneficial consider tests for alternative conditions or specialist referral. Similarly if there is no evidence of airways obstruction following spirometry consider tests for alternative conditions or specialist referral.
- In children with an intermediate probability of asthma who cannot perform spirometry, a trial of treatment should be offered for a specified period; if this is beneficial treat as asthma and arrange a review, if not, stop asthma treatment, consider tests for alternative conditions and specialist referral.

Normal results on testing, especially if performed when the child is asymptomatic, do not exclude a diagnosis of asthma.

## Diagnosis in adults

BTS/SIGN (2014) emphasise that a diagnosis of asthma is made by careful clinical history to determine characteristic pattern of signs and symptoms and a measure of airflow obstruction, preferably via spirometry, where available. Normal spirometry or peak expiratory flow (PEF) measurements made when a person is not symptomatic does not exclude asthma diagnosis. History should also explore possible causes, including occupational. Clinical features that increase the probability of asthma in adults include:

- More than one of the following: wheeze, breathlessness, chest tightness and cough, particularly if symptoms are worse at night/early in the morning, or in response to exercise, allergen exposure or cold air, or after taking aspirin or beta blockers
- History of atopic disorder
- Family history of asthma/atopic disorder
- Widespread wheeze detected on chest auscultation
- Unexplained low forced expiratory volume (FEV1) or PEF
- Unexplained peripheral blood eosinophilia.

(BTS/SIGN 2014)

BTS/SIGN (2014) suggest that following diagnosis, based on assessment of symptoms and measure of airflow obstruction, the following treatment should be instigated:

- Patients with a high probability of asthma should be put straight onto a trial of treatment.
- Patients with a low probability of asthma in whom symptoms are though to point to an alternative diagnosis should be investigated and managed accordingly. Asthma should be reconsidered if no response to treatment.
- In patients with an intermediate probability of asthma further investigations should be carried out, including a trial of treatment before diagnosis is confirmed and maintenance treatment established.

## Chronic obstructive pulmonary disease (COPD)

COPD is characterised by airflow obstruction that is usually progressive, not fully reversible and does not change markedly over several months; diagnosis is based on assessment of signs and symptoms with a measure of severity of airflow obstruction (NICE 2010b). In 2004 NICE published the Thorax guideline: *Management of Chronic Obstructive Pulmonary Disease in Adults in Primary and Secondary Care*, followed by *a partial update* (NICE 2010b) which contains the following recommendations relating to diagnosis.

There is no single diagnostic test for COPD. Diagnosis of COPD relies on clinical judgement based on history, physical examination and confirmation of airflow obstruction using post-bronchodilator spirometry performed by an appropriately trained professional supported by quality control processes and that the skills are available to interpret results. A diagnosis of COPD should be considered in patients over the age of 35 who have a risk factor (generally smoking) and who present with one or more of the following symptoms:

- Exertional breathlessness (graded by the Medical Research Council (MRC) dyspnoea scale)

- Chronic cough
- Regular sputum production
- Frequent winter 'bronchitis'
- Wheeze.

Patients in whom a diagnosis of COPD is considered should also be asked about the presence of the following factors:

- Weight loss
- Effort intolerance
- Waking at night
- Ankle swelling
- Fatigue
- Occupational hazards
- Chest pain or haemoptysis – these are uncommon in COPD and raise the possibility of alternative diagnoses.

(NICE 2010b)

Spirometry should be performed at time of diagnosis and to reconfirm diagnosis where an exceptionally good response to treatment is shown. Drug treatment can be started before diagnosis is confirmed, provided spirometry has been performed and other assessments to exclude asthma have been undertaken. Differential diagnosis of COPD includes any condition that presents with breathlessness or cough. Differentiation between COPD and asthma should be made on the history and clinical examination in untreated patients and on longitudinal observation, PEF and/or spirometry. PEF is not routinely recommended for diagnosis or assessment of people with COPD but may help to distinguish COPD from asthma (NICE 2010b).

## Musculoskeletal conditions

### Arthritis

#### *Osteoarthritis*

Diagnosis of osteoarthritis is usually made following clinical examination and history taking. Pain and restricted function are the main presenting features, prevalence of osteoarthritis of the knee, hip and hand increases with age (CKS 2013c). Osteoarthritis is the most common form of arthritis and refers to a clinical syndrome of joint pain which causes varying degrees of functional limitation and reduces quality of life (NICE 2014e).

Osteoarthritis can be diagnosed clinically without radiological or laboratory investigations if a person is:

- 45 years and over and
- Has activity related joint pain and

- Has either no morning joint related stiffness or morning stiffness that lasts no longer than 30 minutes
- Atypical features such as history of trauma, prolonged morning related stiffness, rapid worsening of symptoms or a hot swollen joint may indicate alternative or additional diagnoses (gout, other inflammatory arthritides, septic arthritis and malignancy).

(NICE 2014e, p.10)

Other key clinical points that can add to diagnostic certainty if required include:

- Gelling – pain and stiffness caused by inactivity. When activity resumes, the pain and stiffness resolve more quickly than with inflammatory types of arthritis (i.e. within 30 minutes)
- Bony swellings and joint deformity
- Crepitus
- Restricted range of joint movement
- Joint tenderness
- Muscle wasting and weakness
- Joint effusions – uncommon except for the knee
- Warmth
- Instability.

(CKS 2013c)

## Rheumatoid arthritis

Diagnosis of rheumatoid arthritis (RA) is based on clinical features and investigations and should be suspected in anyone with persistent synovitis (weeks rather than days) where no other underlying cause is obvious (CKS 2013d). Any person with suspected persistent synovitis of undetermined cause should be referred for specialist opinion, with urgent referral if any of the following apply:

- Small joints of the hand or feet are affected
- More than one joint is affected
- There has been a delay of three months or longer between onset of symptoms and seeking medical advice.

(NICE 2009c)

Typical clinical features of synovitis include pain, swelling and heat in affected joints with stiffness often worse in the morning and after inactivity, usually lasting more than 30 minutes. Symptoms can be accompanied by rheumatoid nodules, systemic features of malaise, fatigue, fever, sweats and weight loss. RA can present as gradual onset, although some people have a rapid, relapsing and remitting course. Symmetrical swelling and tenderness of the small joints of the hands and feet are usually found on examination, although any synovial joint can be affected (CKS 2013d).

There is no specific diagnostic test and all people with suspected RA should be referred for specialist assessment. Investigations are not necessary in primary care but the following tests can speed up the diagnostic process and act as baseline prior to treatment: C-reactive protein (CRP) or erythrocyte sedimentation rate (ESR), full blood count, liver function tests, urea and electrolytes, rheumatoid factor, antinuclear antibodies, radiology, ultrasound or MRI. Investigations should not delay referral for suspected RA (CKS 2013c).

## Osteoporosis

The following information relating to diagnosis of osteoporosis is provided by CKS (2013a). Osteoporosis is a disease characterised by low bone mass and structural deterioration of bone tissue, resulting in subsequent increase in bone fragility and susceptibility to fracture, it is asymptomatic and usually undiagnosed until a fragility fracture occurs. Fragility fractures are defined as fractures following a fall from standing height or less, although can occur spontaneously, they can occur in the wrist, spine and hip but also in the arm, pelvis, ribs and other bones (CKS 2013a).

CKS (2013a) state the following:

> Osteoporosis is defined by the World Health Organisation as a bone mineral density (BMD) of 2.5 standard deviations below the mean peak mass (average of young healthy adults) as measured by dual-energy X-ray absorptiometry (DEXA) applied to the femoral neck and reported as a T-score. However, BMD measurement does not assess the structural deterioration in bone and consequently, most osteoporotic fractures occur in women who do not have osteoporosis as defined by a T-score equal to or less than –2.5.

Both the National Osteoporosis Guideline Group (NOGG) and NICE provide separate and different guidance on when and how to assess osteoporotic fracture risk and it is therefore recommended that the reader accesses the CKS site where a summary of the key point from each guidance can be read, prior to deciding which to use (CKS 2013a).

## Conclusion

This chapter has provided an overview of diagnostic criteria and the signs and symptoms associated with many, but by no means all, of the LTCs that often present in primary care. Although for some of these diagnosis will be made and treatment plans instigated in primary care, other LTCs will require more specialist input to ensure a correct diagnosis is made. No diagnosis should be made without taking a clear history and conducting an appropriate clinical examination.

## Key points

- Diagnosis of an LTC should always include careful history taking and clinical examination.
- Where diagnostic criteria exist these should be interpreted with regard to the overall clinical picture, for many LTCs negative investigations do not necessarily rule out positive diagnosis.
- Differential diagnosis should always be considered, particularly where signs and symptoms vary, or if improvement is not achieved with an appropriate treatment plan.
- Diagnosis for some LTCs can be complex and referral to specialists for firm diagnosis should be made where recommended in the guidelines.

## Further areas to consider

- Which conditions should be referred for specialist investigation?
- Are you aware of the relevant referral procedures in your area?
- Which evidence-based sources are you aware of where you can access diagnostic criteria?
- How do you ensure that you have the relevant skills for history taking/ clinical examination?

<table>
<tr><td>7</td><td>

# Effective management of people with a long-term condition

</td></tr>
</table>

---

### Overview

This chapter provides a practical guide on clinical management including issues such as: writing a protocol, registration, recall and review, follow-up appointments, referral criteria and quality assurance mechanisms. Ways of identifying patients in the practice population to ensure registers are up to date are discussed, including how to ensure an effective call/recall system.

---

## Introduction

So far national and international policies guiding the care and management of people with long-term conditions (LTCs) have been reviewed, along with the key principles relating to care provision, including case management and the importance of self-care. The physical and psychological aspects of living with an LTC have been discussed along with social influences on health. The key principles of behaviour change and motivational interviewing have been introduced and examples provided of how to put these principles into practice. In Chapter 6 signs, symptoms and criteria relating to diagnosis were introduced to ensure that people with LTCs are identified. The importance of IT systems, the use of shared records and the benefits of assistive technology should also not be forgotten. So what next you may ask? Once diagnosis is established and the type and level of care provision have been determined how do you actually implement all this? How can you ensure that the service you provide to people with LTCs runs smoothly and efficiently, that care is not duplicated or essential elements missed and that people are not lost to review? The aim of this chapter is to discuss the practicalities involved in day-to-day management of people with an LTC in primary care and encourage you to start thinking about the service you currently provide, how can you make it better?

## Protocols

The words protocol, protocol-based care and protocol-based services feature in many of the UK guiding government policies, particularly in the National Service Frameworks (NSFs). Indeed they were considered an integral part of the Department of Health (DH) NHS plan which stated:

> By 2004 the majority of NHS will be working under agreed protocols identifying how common conditions should be handled and which staff can best handle them. The new NHS Modernisation Agency will lead a major drive to ensure that protocol-based care takes hold throughout the NHS. It will work with the National Institute for Clinical Excellence, patients, clinicians and managers to develop clear protocols that make the best use of all the talents of NHS staff and which are flexible enough to take account of patients' individual needs.
>
> (DH 2000b, p.83)

The NHS Institute for Innovation and Improvement, now administered by NHS Quality, notes that protocol-based care enables NHS staff to put evidence into practice by determining what should be done, when, where and by whom at a local level, providing a framework for multi-disciplinary teams. Furthermore they note that local protocols provide descriptions of the steps taken to care for and treat a patient, they can also be referred to as 'integrated care pathways', 'patient group directions' and 'referral advice'. They normally include decision support systems about appropriate care for specific clinical circumstances, forming all or part of the record of care. Rycroft-Malone et al. (2009, p.1490) suggest: 'protocol-based care can be viewed as a mechanism for facilitating standardisation of care and streamlining decision-making through rationalising the information with which to make judgements and ultimately decisions'.

Protocols have long been used in the primary care setting to guide practice, define the roles of the health care professionals and provide a guide to all those involved with the day-to-day practicalities of care provision.

A protocol should:

- Be an agreed strategy for carrying out a procedure or activity
- Be evidence based but reflect local need
- Form a structured framework to prevent duplication of services and maintain standards amongst all team members
- Identify clear roles of responsibility for all those involved
- Be an integral part of the audit cycle, evaluating patient care.

So what sort of practical issues should be included in a protocol for people with LTCs? Box 7.1 provides a guide to the general areas that should be addressed within a protocol.

## Box 7.1    Protocol

- Register – who maintains and updates it
- Recall system – computer or paper based?
- Identification of a system to recall people who do not attend (DNA)
- General administration issues (who will be responsible for sending review/recall letters, what system will be put in place to ensure that they are informed if someone DNAs or can't attend an appointment?)
- Timing of clinic/appointment (will it suit the client need – are this client group of working age, would an early morning/evening clinic appointment be more appropriate?)
- Timing of appointments (how long is required – need to consider newly diagnosed, routine review and annual review)
- Location
- Resources required (for clinical issues e.g. Doppler for peripheral arterial disease (PAD) assessment, tuning fork for diabetic foot assessment, spirometer for respiratory review and supportive literature e.g. peak flow/blood glucose monitoring diaries, literature related to self-help groups, condition-specific leaflets etc.)
- How often should review take place (six monthly/annually)?
- What will be incorporated into the review? (Routine and annual)
- Roles of each health care professional e.g. health care assistant (HCA), registered nurse, GP, dietitian, podiatrist, pharmacist etc.
- Educational needs of each health care professional involved (e.g. if HCA to take blood pressure, who teaches them that skill? Would clinic be improved if the registered nurse providing the care has an independent prescribing qualification, has the GP attended regular updates to ensure their knowledge is up to date regarding the LTCs they are responsible for?)
- Physical parameters to be measured: height/weight/body mass index (BMI)/blood tests/blood pressure/urinalysis etc.
- Which, if any, of these physical parameters need to be performed prior to the review appointment so results are available at review?
- Type of physical/clinical examination to be performed and by whom?
- Medication review
- Type of psychological assessment to be performed and by whom?
- Education – for both the person with the LTC, their family and carers, what needs to be included e.g. advice re driving, restricted occupations, self-care
- Available local initiatives e.g. Expert Patients Programme (EPP)
- Referral criteria – both within the team and outside the team
- Audit – how will the quality of the care provided be measured?
- Protocol review date – at least yearly, or earlier if new evidence dictates.

**Box 7.2   Example of areas that could be included in an annual structured review for an adult with epilepsy**

- Information should be provided to the person with epilepsy and their family/carers
- The following should be discussed: (i) Seizure control (ii) Any adverse effects of medication (iii) Concordance with current medication
- If seizure control is inadequate: (i) ensure medication is being taken correctly as prescribed (ii) specialist advice should be sought, or a referral made, before medication is changed (iii) epilepsy specialist nurses are good resources to discuss any issues identified within the review
- Ask about how epilepsy is affecting the person's daily functioning and quality of life, including work, education and leisure activities
- Assess for symptoms of anxiety or depression
- It should be ascertained that all people with epilepsy have (i) an accessible point of contact with specialist services (ii) a comprehensive care plan is in place (iii) access to an epilepsy specialist nurse
- Regular blood test monitoring is not recommended unless clinically indicated (e.g. suspected toxicity, adjustment of phenytoin dose)
- Blood tests for: full blood count (fbc), electrolytes, liver enzymes, vitamin D and other test of bone metabolism should be performed 2–5 yearly in adult taking enzyme-inducing drugs.

(adapted from CKS 2014b)

**Box 7.3   Example of an annual structured review for an adult with type 2 diabetes**

- At least one week prior to review (to ensure results available for discussion at review): HbA1c (glycated haemoglobin), urea and electrolytes (including serum creatinine), eGFR, liver function tests, full lipid screen, thyroid function tests, early morning urine for albumin:creatinine ratio (in the absence of proteinurea/urinary tract infection)
- Blood pressure
- BMI/waist measurement
- Examine patient's feet and lower legs to detect risk factors – include: testing of foot sensation using 10g microfilament or vibration, palpation of foot pulses, inspection for foot deformity, inspection of footwear; agree management plan including footcare education, or refer if indicated by assessment
- Ask about neuropathic symptoms e.g. foot problems, erectile dysfunction, gastroparesis

*(continued)*

*(continued)*

- Individual ongoing nutritional advice should be given by a health care professional with specific expertise
- Discussion of self-monitoring of blood glucose, where appropriate
- Ongoing structured patient education should be offered to the person with diabetes, their family and carers
- Discussion of lifestyle issues e.g. smoking cessation, exercise
- Structured screening for depression
- Ensure structured eye surveillance has been performed (ideally through quality assured retinal photography programme)
- Review cardiovascular risk
- Medication review.

(adapted from NICE 2009b)

Box 7.4 includes general recommendations (taken from CKS 2013a) relating to the type of issues that could be included in a review of a patient with osteoporosis.

---

### Box 7.4    Potential areas to include in a review of a patient with osteoporosis

- Education regarding disease process and importance of intervention therapies
- Medication review – concordance with current therapy/review of any side effects
- Pain assessment
- Any falls since last review?
- Discussion (to include family/carers as appropriate) re interventions to prevent falls; i.e. modifying home environment, modifying living habits (such as wearing of appropriate footwear), installing appropriate aids (handrails, non slip bathmat), modifying medications that may predispose to falls, correction of poor vision, referral to appropriate support services
- Discussion re lifestyle factors e.g. weight, smoking, alcohol
- Advice re exercise programmes including high intensity strength training and low impact weight bearing exercise
- For people taking oral corticosteroids, continue treatment with bisphosphonates at least until they stop treatment with corticosteroids.
- For people not taking oral corticosteroids, review the need for continuing treatment with bisphosphonates after five years
- For people who remain at high risk of an osteoporotic fracture, continue treatment without further assessment
- If repeat DXA scanning is thought to be appropriate, in general this should not be carried out unless the person has been taking treatment for at least two years

- Repeat DXA scanning should be considered if a woman has another fragility fracture despite adhering fully to treatment with a bisphosphonate for one year.

(CKS 2013a)

## Evidence supporting the 3 Rs

The benefits of organisational interventions to improve recall and review, in addition to multifaceted interventions to improve the performance of practitioners in enhancing the care of people with diabetes, have been previously demonstrated in two Cochrane systematic reviews (Griffin and Kinmonth 2000; Renders et al. 2001). This was further supported by a large randomised controlled trial (RCT) in Denmark (Olivarius et al. 2001) that randomised GPs to a control and intervention group. The intervention group were given patient leaflets, guidelines, annual seminars and feedback, prompted to review patients, encouraged to set and subsequently revise realistic treatment goals and exposed to a charismatic opinion leader. Additional interventions to improve care of diabetes in the community included patient education and support for self-management, changes in delivery systems such as enhancement of the involvement of nurses, and additional decision support for practitioners. Results indicated statistically significant improvements in both glycated haemoglobin and blood pressure, with subsequent observed risk reductions in cardiovascular and microvascular complications. Griffin (2001) noted that caution should be taken in interpreting the results, in that the recruited GPs were particularly motivated, further noting that many primary care teams outside of these research studies fail to achieve the same intensive management of multiple risk factors. He emphasises that once the 3 Rs are firmly established what is it that makes the difference? Was it the setting and reassessment of personalised, realistic goals by practitioners, congruent with evidence from psychology, or that patients who received the intervention are more actively involved in their care, more satisfied, and more likely to adhere to medication than those in routine care? Whatever the reasons behind the improved health outcomes it is important that practitioners take the message from studies such as these on board and review the way they provide care to maximise overall health outcomes for all people with LTCs.

Fahey et al. (2006) conducted a Cochrane systematic review relating to people with hypertension with two key objectives:

1. To determine the effectiveness of interventions to improve control of blood pressure in patients with hypertension.
2. To evaluate the effectiveness of reminders on improving the follow-up of patients with hypertension.

Similar results were seen as in previous reviews. Fifty-six RCTs met the inclusion criteria, six types of interventions were reviewed including: self-monitoring, educational interventions directed to the patient, educational interventions directed to the health professional, health professional (nurse or pharmacist) led care, organisational interventions that aimed to improve the delivery of care, appointment reminder systems. Results did vary according to each intervention. Self-monitoring was associated with moderate net reduction in diastolic blood pressure and appointment reminders increased the proportion of individuals who attended for follow-up. Educational interventions directed at patients or health professionals, however, appeared unlikely to be associated with large net reductions in blood pressure. Health professional (nurse or pharmacist) led care appeared to be a promising way of delivering care but requires further evaluation. Fahey et al. (2006) concluded that despite the variability of methodological quality and the heterogeneous results from RCTs related to some of the interventions, an organised system of regular follow-up and review, combined with a vigorous stepped care approach to antihypertensive drug treatment, appeared to be the most likely way to improve the control of high blood pressure.

In relation to epilepsy Redhead (2003) noted that despite epilepsy being the most common serious neurological disorder in the UK, a lack of neurologists means that patients' day-to-day prescribing, supervision and support often depends on primary care. He suggested that an improvement in the process of care in the primary care setting can result from three important strategies:

> appropriately trained practice nurses running practice nurse-led clinics; structured management of care, through registration, which facilitates audit, prescription monitoring, and recall; and, finally, improved teamwork and communication based on protocols locally agreed upon between primary and secondary care.
>
> (Redhead 2003, p.54)

There is evidence that structured programmes of care with efficient registration and recall systems have a positive effect on health outcomes and in most areas there is always room for improvement. This was clearly demonstrated in the 2008 Improvement Foundation's National Primary Care Collaborative Programme, which prior to the implementation of the GMS contract (BMA/NHS Confederation 2003) set up a programme to help GP practices to achieve improvements for patients with established cardiovascular disease (CVD) – secondary prevention. Later phases of the programme included diabetes and chronic obstructive pulmonary disease (COPD). The aim of the work was to ensure that patients received optimum care through the application of a systematic, sustainable approach. The improvements demonstrated by the programme in improving the management of LTCs was later incorporated into the QOF. The collaborative worked with practices asking them to focus their efforts around a number of key principles:

* Know all your patients who have coronary heart disease (CHD)
* Be systematic and proactive in managing care
* Ensure timely and high quality support from secondary care
* Involve patients in delivering and developing care
* Develop effective links with other key local partners.

(Improvement Foundation 2008)

Case studies demonstrating how practices improved their care included developing practice agreed protocols, telephone reminders to non-attenders, sending practice nurses on a validated training programme to enable them to run enhanced CHD clinics and holding educational events for GPs run by the local cardiologist, amongst other initiatives. Overall results of the CHD secondary prevention programme, which included a total of 5,442 general practices, indicated a fourfold reduction in mortality for patients with CHD in participating Primary Care Trusts (PCTs) compared to non-participants. This was equivalent to 3,000 lives from myocardial infarctions (MI) saved per year and a reduction of non-fatal MI by 3,000 per year. The Improvement Foundation state that they have improved the care of LTCs across thousands of practices in England, Scotland, Canada and Australia.

However it is worth ending this section with a word of caution. In the past ten years work in the UK with regard to improving organisational structure in relation to LTC management has been mainly focused around the QOF. Much has been written about the negative, as well as the positive impact of standardisation of practice (for example see Timmermans and Berg 2003; Scott et al. 2011), particularly through financially incentivised organisational interventions such as the QOF. A systematic review undertaken by Gillam et al. (2012), for example on the impact of the QOF on primary care concluded that both doctors and nurses believed that the person-centeredness of consultations and continuity were negatively affected, although they also argue that nurses have reported enhanced specialist skills since the implementation of the QOF. Indeed my own research (Carrier 2014) has indicated that practice nurses are generally enthusiastic towards the standardisation imposed by the QOF which has allowed them to increase their autonomy within the 'safety net' provided by the structured review the QOF promotes. Whilst the QOF has incentivised general practice to have a more organised approach to LTC management, full use has not always been made of disease registers and there has been limited evidence of the direct impact of the QOF on improving public health or reducing health inequalities and evidence as to whether the QOF has influenced improvements in clinical care is equivocal (Dixon et al. 2011). Dixon et al. (2011, p.5) suggest that: 'The QOF has promoted a medicalised and mechanistic approach to managing chronic disease, which does not support holistic, patient-centred care, or promote self-care and self-management'.

Structuring care in a systematic way to encourage regular review is clearly important but practitioners also need to consider the type of care they provide and continue to provide individualised patient-centred care that recognises co-morbidities, health and social care needs and promotes self-care and self-management.

## Teamwork and referral criteria

As teams develop and the concept of skill mix in health care delivery becomes an increasingly more popular concept in primary care the importance of referral criteria and a clear awareness of each other's roles becomes even more important. The benefits of a multi-disciplinary approach and the importance of teamwork have been discussed in Chapter 3, but within the primary health care setting an awareness of the roles of all those involved, including the patient and carer is essential. A team approach to care can improve accessibility for people with LTCs and expand the range of services offered. Clear referral criteria should however be built into the protocol to ensure that each team member is aware of their limitations and is aware of when it is appropriate to seek more specialised advice. Clear channels of communication should be established and maintained to ensure that people referred to other members of the team are seen quickly and by the most appropriate person.

## Quality improvement and audit

Monitoring and evaluation of all services provided should be considered an integral part of protocol development, through the process of clinical audit, an essential element of quality improvement. Clinical audit has been defined as: 'The systematic and critical analysis of the quality of clinical care, a quality improvement process that seeks to improve patient care and outcomes through systematic review of care against explicit criteria and the implementation of change' (NICE 2002).

Clinical audit was considered a central feature of the clinical governance umbrella (Box 7.5), an organisational approach to quality initially introduced in the UK as a response to concerns about quality of health care in the NHS, most notably the Bristol inquiry, a public inquiry into children's heart surgery in the Bristol Royal Infirmary 1984–1995. Clinical governance was first defined in the DH (1998) consultation document *A First Class Service: Quality in the New NHS* as: 'A framework through which NHS organisations are accountable for continuously improving the quality of their services and safeguarding high standards of care by creating an environment in which excellence in clinical care will flourish.'

---

### Box 7.5   The clinical governance umbrella

The clinical governance umbrella consisted of a number of key components including:

- Patient, public and carer involvement
- Risk management – incident reporting, infection control, prevention and control of risk
- Staff management and performance – recruitment, workforce planning, appraisals
- Education, training and continuous professional development
- Clinical audit management, planning and monitoring, learning through research and audit
- Information management
- Communication – patient and public, external partners, internal, board and organisation-wide
- Leadership
- Team working.

(DH 1998)

---

**Table 7.1 Key features that distinguish clinical audits from research**

| Research | Audit |
|---|---|
| Discovers the right thing to do | Determines whether the right thing is being done |
| A series of 'one-off' projects | A cyclical series of reviews |
| Collects complex data | Collects routine data |
| Experiment rigorously defined | Review of what clinicians actually do |
| Often possible to generalise the findings | Not possible to generalise from the findings |

The NHS in Wales (2012) have more recently defined governance as: 'A system of accountability to citizens, service users, stakeholders and the wider community, within which health care organisations work, take decisions and lead their people to achieve their objectives.'

The aim of clinical audit is to: assess and improve quality of care, act as an aid to continuing professional development, provide individuals and teams with a sense of both personal and professional achievement and assess what you are doing and whether you can make it better. One of the recommendations of the Bristol Inquiry was that clinical audit should be at the core of a system of local monitoring of performance and should be compulsory for all health care professionals providing clinical care. When conducted well, clinical audit provides a way in which quality of care can be reviewed objectively within a supportive and developmental culture. Audit has a number of well-documented key features that clearly distinguish it from research which have been reproduced in a number of audit training manuals, these are outlined in Table 7.1.

Clinical audit is about getting it right, ensuring the service you provide is evidence-based, effective and meets the need of the people at whom it is aimed. Since the introduction of the QOF many of the clinical targets relating to LTCs are included in a regular audit programme, for example:

- The percentage of patients on the diabetes register who have a HbA1c recorded
- The percentage of patients on the chronic kidney disease (CKD) register with hypertension and proteinuria who are treated with an angiotensin converting enzyme inhibitor (ACE) or angiotensin receptor blocker (ARB).

However audit should also include quality issues such as people's perception of the type of service offered and whether it meets their needs. The key stages of audit (Figure 7.1) include:

1. Selection of topic
2. Decide on element of care or activity to be measured – criteria (e.g. HbA1c) and set an appropriate and realistic standard (e.g. 85 per cent of all people on diabetes register)
3. Collect data
4. Evaluate findings, assess performance against criteria and standard

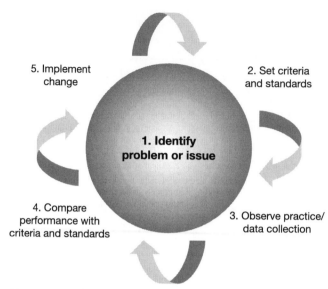

**Figure 7.1** The audit cycle

5.  Act to make improvements, making any relevant changes identified as required
6.  Repeat data collection, evaluation and take further action if required.

It is vital to always close the audit loop by setting a date when the service will be re-audited to ensure improvements are made or maintained.

The four UK countries continue to build on previous quality improvement initiatives, including building on the initial principles of clinical governance, in order to continue to deliver sustainable and continuous quality improvement of both health and social care systems (Royal College of Nursing (RCN) 2014). Continuous improvement of the quality, effectiveness and safety of health services and the patient experience are enshrined in the NHS Mandate in England (DH 2013a) with the focus on improving health and care outcomes. In Wales the focus is on quality improvement methodologies including national audit and outcomes reviews, a patient safety programme and methodologies for improvement and audit developed by 1000 Lives Plus (NHS Wales 2013). Northern Ireland has a ten-year strategy and implementation plan, focusing on the six dimensions of quality health care (safe; effective; patient-centred; timely; efficient; equitable) (Department of Health, Social Services and Public Safety (DHSSPSNI) 2012a); these six dimensions are also central to the Quality Strategy for NHS Scotland (2013). The reader is advised to consider what quality initiatives are taking place in your own country and how this impacts on your individual practice.

## Telehealth and telecare

Telehealth is defined as: 'The remote exchange of data between a patient at home and their clinician(s) to assist in diagnosis and monitoring typically used to support patients with Long Term Conditions' (Telecare Services Association 2013).

Telehealth uses technology to assist people with the management of LTCs, enabling them to take control over their own health, monitoring information about their health condition to identify health issues before they become critical. Telehealth works through monitoring vital signs and transmitting these to a centre or health care professional to be monitored against set parameters (Telecare Services Association 2013).

Telecare is defined as: 'Support and assistance provided at a distance using information and communication technology. It is the continuous, automatic and remote monitoring of users by means of sensors to enable them to continue living in their own home' (Telecare Services Association 2013).

A systematic review on telehealth from the King's Fund (2012) identified 64 studies across seven different health conditions that measured the impact of telehealth; the majority of these looked at diabetes, heart failure and stroke. Results included a reduction in hospitalisation from heart failure related to remote monitoring, positive reduction in HbA1c from patients needing intensive insulin therapy transmitting self-monitored blood glucose results. Overall results were less positive for multiple rather than single LTCs. Online support tools were found to have a positive impact in patients with depression. Studies of hypertension management were positive in terms of clinical effectiveness and patient-reported outcomes. Positive benefits were shown on the impact of telehealth in reducing hospital admissions from COPD, although results on clinical effectiveness and care experience were mixed. The King's Fund website provides access to a number of publications related to telecare and telehealth. As this is an area that is being constantly updated the reader is advised to access this information at: www.kingsfund.org.uk/topics/telecare-and-telehealth. Additional information is available from the Telecare and telehealth reading room: www.kingsfund.org.uk/topics/telecare-and-telehealth/library.

## Rehabilitation and palliative (end of life) care

Finally two other important areas to consider when designing individual care plans for people with LTCs are rehabilitation and palliative care. Whilst it is not in the remit of this book to explore these in detail (both are book subjects in their own right) brief mention is made here of schemes that have been developed to support people in maximising their life opportunities in the context of their condition(s) or in supporting both patients and carers at the end of life. Readers interested or working in these areas are encouraged to access further texts and resources aimed at exploring both topics in greater depth.

## Rehabilitation

Within the UK much work has been done on the development of cardiac and pulmonary rehabilitation programmes. Schemes such as these generally involve programmes of exercise and information sessions to support people in returning to their everyday activities successfully. They provide both physical and psychological support for patients and their families. See:

British Heart Foundation – cardiac rehabilitation: www.bhf.org.uk/heart-health/living-with-a-heart-condition/cardiac-rehabilitation

British Thoracic Society – pulmonary rehabilitation: www.brit-thoracic.org.uk/guidelines-and-quality-standards/pulmonary-rehabilitation-guideline/

Rehabilitation schemes focus on multi-disciplinary team involvement using a variety of therapeutic interventions to restore both patients' functional abilities and improve quality of life.

---

**Pause for reflection**

What rehabilitation schemes are available in your area for people with LTCs?

Draw up a list of available schemes and find out what these programmes involve, so you can advise patients what to expect.

If you can, arrange to join in a session to allow you to experience for yourself the challenges faced by people with LTCs.

---

## Palliative (end of life) care

The World Health Organisation (WHO 1990, p.11) defines palliative care as:

> The active total care of patients whose disease is not responsive to curative treatment. Control of pain, of other symptoms and of psychological, social and physical problems is paramount.
>
> The goal of palliative care is achievement of the best quality of life for patients and their families.

End of life care focuses on the support of people approaching death, enabling them to die with dignity and additionally supports their family and carers (NHS Choices 2014). It can involve a number of health and social care professionals and the care provided is irrespective of the condition leading to end of life. Patients are considered to be approaching the end of life when they are likely to die within the next 12 months, but it can also include patients who are anticipated to die within a few days or hours, those with life-threatening conditions caused by a sudden catastrophic event or people who are frail and have co-existing conditions (NHS Choices 2014).

---

**Pause for reflection**

Are you involved in caring for people at the end of life?

Do you feel adequately prepared to provide support for patients at the end of life and their family/carers?

A number of specific educational programmes and resources are available for health care professionals who may be providing end of life care and readers are encouraged to ensure that they are themselves adequately prepared to provide support to patients, their family and carers.

## Conclusion

This chapter has addressed many of the practical issues relating to providing systematic and structured care to people with LTCs in the primary care environment, including brief mention of the services offered by telehealth/telecare and a very brief introduction to rehabilitation and palliative (end of life) care. Readers interested in, or providing services in these areas should ensure they access further information and educational programmes that address these issues in further depth. It is recommended that PHCTs review the services they provide and ensure that systems are in place to review all patients with LTCs incorporating both generic principles of care and condition-specific elements and develop individualised care plans that focus on health promotion and supported self-care. Regardless of the type of LTC, structured protocols, developed by all the team members who are to be involved in the care provision, should be developed and regularly updated, either annually or as new evidence dictates. Quality criteria should be built into the protocol to ensure that the service provided is meeting the needs of people with LTCs.

## Key points

- Structured organisational interventions such as regular follow-up and review and appointment reminders improve overall health outcomes for people with LTCs and should be used to support development of individualised care plans.
- Regularly updated protocols can be used as a team building exercise and also to identify educational needs of team members.
- Clinical audit criteria and standards should be considered an integral part of protocol development.
- Standardisation should not negatively impact individualised person-centred care.

## Further areas to consider

- Are structured protocols in place for LTCs in your practice area, do they address all conditions?

- Do you meet regularly as a team to discuss new evidence that may have an impact on effective health care delivery?
- Who is responsible for ensuring that local protocols are updated and reflect recent evidence?
- Does each team member understand each other's role and when it is appropriate to refer to another team member?
- How do you ensure you are consistently monitoring and improving the quality of care you provide?
- Have you received adequate educational preparation for the roles you are involved in?

well-built question should have three or four elements. For example, in the 'PICO' method, recommended by the NHS Executive (1999), the key elements are:

- Problem
- Intervention
- Comparison (if required)
- Outcome.

The focus of the question may be diagnosis, prognosis, a health care intervention or the cost effectiveness or efficiency of an intervention (NHS Executive 1999). The PICO method can be used to translate initial thoughts about a gap between evidence and practice into an answerable question. For example, a question such as: 'What is the best method to teach adults diagnosed with asthma, to help them recognise the signs of an asthma exacerbation?' could be translated into four parts using the PICO method (Box 8.1). Framing the question in this way makes it possible not only to think harder about the individual aspects of the problem, and what you actually need to know, but also helps define the search terms, which is important for database searching.

---

## Box 8.1  The PICO method

What is the best method to teach adults diagnosed with asthma, to help them recognise the signs of an asthma exacerbation?

**Problem:** In adults diagnosed with asthma
**Intervention:** What are the benefits of teaching regular peak flow measurement
**Comparison:** Instead of, or in addition to, teaching recognition of deteriorating asthma through identification of specific symptoms?
**Outcome:** In recognising the signs of an asthma exacerbation and reducing the overall incidence of emergency consultations/admissions.

---

Not all questions will relate to research studies that use quantitative methods. For example a question such as 'What methods do adults diagnosed with asthma in primary care feel are most helpful in recognising early signs of an asthma exacerbation?' would be better answered by studies utilising qualitative methods of inquiry. To answer questions that involve finding out the person or carer's viewpoint on a particular intervention, or to gain understanding about a condition from their perspective, the PICO method can still be used or a different acronym may be useful to answer the question. The SPICE acronym (Box 8.2) includes the following elements:

- Setting
- Perspective
- (Area) of Interest, Intervention or Interpretation
- Context or Comparison (if required)
- Evaluation.

---

**Box 8.2   The SPICE acronym**

What methods do adults diagnosed with asthma in primary care feel are most helpful in recognising early signs of an asthma exacerbation?

**Setting:** Primary care
**Perspective:** Of adults diagnosed with asthma
**(Area) of Interest:** The usefulness of methods used to assist in recognising early signs of an asthma exacerbation
**Comparison:** Instead of, or in addition to, teaching recognition of deteriorating asthma through identification of specific symptoms?
**Evaluation:** Methods adults with asthma feel are most helpful in recognising early signs of an asthma exacerbation.

---

**Pause for reflection**

Think of a problem that you have come across, relating to LTC management, where you were not sure of the evidence base and phrase it into an answerable question using the PICO or SPICE method.

## Searching for evidence

The third step, searching for the evidence, is one that nurses and other health care professionals often find the most difficult. A search of large databases such as the Current Index to Nursing and Allied Health Literature (CINAHL) or PubMed (publicly available MEDLINE) can be time consuming and frustrating for inexperienced users, who, because of a lack of knowledge of advanced searching techniques, may either find vast amounts of inappropriate information or, alternatively, may miss essential information. For a busy nurse working in primary care, who needs to find information quickly, such databases may appear daunting. Librarians and information specialists can support you in developing systematic searching skills. There are systems in place in databases such PubMed to help retrieve high-quality articles. It is not possible to go into precise detail within the limits of this chapter, but Bidwell (2004) provides a comprehensive guide to searching PubMed, using features such as the 'clinical queries' mode, which can assist in reducing the volume of information often obtained when performing a simple search. Most databases such as PubMed provide their own online tutorials, unique to each database, which are quick and easy to access and follow.

**Pause for reflection**

Are you skilled in database searching or have you ever experienced frustration when trying to find an answer? Think about what databases you have accessed and whether you have had any difficulties with searching, do you find too much, or too little information? Have you had instruction in database searching or accessed online tutorials?

## Critical appraisal

Once the evidence has been found, the fourth step is critical appraisal, which can also prove difficult for those with limited time. A number of appraisal tools are available to assist practitioners in appraising primary evidence, for example the Critical Appraisal Skills Programme (CASP) tools and checklists (www.casp-uk.net/#!casp-tools-check lists/c18f8) and JBI Critical Appraisal Tools. Fortunately, there are also easy ways to access information that has been subjected to a variety of forms of critical review. A question may already have been asked and the answer may be available in a critically appraised study, but the key is in knowing where to look. The first thing to know is that research exists in two forms: primary evidence (e.g. RCTs, cohort studies, case control studies, qualitative studies) and evaluated or secondary resources (systematic reviews, meta-analyses, clinical guidelines, narrative or meta-synthesis, critical reviews, query answering services) (Bidwell 2004). It can be time consuming to sift though primary evidence and sometimes studies can be contradictory, more accessible research reports can exaggerate the effects of interventions. Secondary (evaluated) sources aim to track down all information, including that which may be inaccessible to practitioners. This information is then appraised using robust methods.

Systematic reviews and meta-analyses are considered the 'gold standard' of evidence for quantitative (positivist) research, because they use explicit criteria to identify and appraise all the literature on a particular topic (NHS Executive 1999). Systematic reviews of evidence favour meta-analysis of RCTs, considered 'gold standard' in trials of effectiveness (cause and effect), with other quantitative methods ranked lower in terms of effectiveness. Narrative synthesis and meta-synthesis have been developed as methods to combine findings from qualitative (naturalistic) research, mixed methods studies or quantitative studies where a statistical approach to combining findings is not necessarily the best method (Centre for Reviews and Dissemination (CRD) 2009; Joanna Briggs Institute (JBI) 2014). These methods appreciate that whilst RCTs are the best methods in answering 'cause and effect' questions, interpretive and qualitative research methods are more appropriate in studies aimed at exploring and interpreting experiences and gaining a more in-depth understanding of human behaviour.

Good quality guidelines and critical reviews will have used a comprehensive search strategy to track down all the evidence on a specific topic and will have used a robust critical appraisal tool to determine their overall findings and recommendations. High calibre guidelines should provide advice to practitioners based on the best evidence available and will utilise systematic reviews, where available, to develop these recommendations. Critical literature reviews can vary in quality, depending on the search strategy utilised, and can be biased towards the author's opinion if limited literature is accessed. A third source of evidence is query answering services, which provide a valuable service to busy practitioners. They conduct 'quick and dirty' searches, which although not of the same standard as systematic reviews, utilise established quality criteria and point practitioners in the right direction of available evidence. They too utilise systematic reviews and high calibre guidelines, where available, to provide an answer, but will also provide brief critical appraisal and summaries of other sources of evidence in areas where less substantial bodies of evidence are obtainable.

For those wishing to learn more about critical appraisal Trisha Greenhalgh's (2014) book *How to Read a Paper* is essential reading. In addition to this there are many organisations that provide training in critical skills appraisal such as CASP that provides workshops and learning resources, including appraisal tools to provide individuals and organisations with the skills on which to base not only their clinical practice, but also policy and decision-making, on robust evidence of effectiveness.

### Pause for reflection

Have you ever changed your practice based on a headline-hitting article that you found when browsing through the latest clinical journals, or do you always seek out further supportive information before altering your practice?

## Finding reliable secondary (evaluated) sources

### UK portals

A number of sites provide access to evaluated high-quality information. Accessing these sites first can reduce searching time and also ensure that the information found is both of high quality and has been subjected to regular updating in light of new evidence. Within the UK NHS websites provide free and easy access to evidence-based sites that were previously restricted to subscribers (Box 8.3). All NHS staff, or those caring for NHS patients, are able to apply for a password, which allows access to numerous sites otherwise limited to subscribers.

---

### Box 8.3    UK NHS websites

National Institute for Health and Care Excellence (NICE) – Evidence Search Health and Social Care (England): www.evidence.nhs.uk/

Health in Wales e-library: www.wales.nhs.uk/researchandresources/elibrary

Health on the Net Northern Ireland (HONNI): www.honni.qub.ac.uk

NHS Scotland – The Knowledge Network: www.knowledge.scot.nhs.uk/home. aspx

## Accessing systematic reviews, meta-analysis and narrative synthesis

One of the best-known sources of both primary and secondary (evaluated) sources of evidence is the Cochrane Library, which consists of a collection of regularly updated databases of evidence. A number of countries provide free access to the Cochrane Library for health care professionals through funded provision, including: all countries of the UK, Australia, New Zealand, Ireland, Denmark, Finland, Norway, Spain, India, parts of Canada, Wyoming in the USA, Latin America and the Caribbean, sponsored South African residents and over 100 low- and middle-income countries (details correct at time of going to press, June 2015; for further details see Cochrane Library website (Box 8.5)). It is considered to be the first resource for information about the effects of health care interventions and includes the Database of Abstracts of Reviews of Effects (DARE), the Health Technology Assessment (HTA) and the NHS Economic Evaluation Database (EED), which can also be accessed directly from the website of the CRD at the University of York (Box 8.4). National Institute for Health Research funding to produce DARE and NHS EED ceased at the end of March 2015 (for further information see the CRD website (Box 8.5)).

CRD also provide a range of other services including an enquiry service that searches its databases for an answer to a question, a helpdesk for searching the databases and information resources page. Other key sources of systematic reviews include the Berkeley Systematic Review Group in the USA and the aforementioned Australia-based Joanna Briggs Institute (Box 8.5). JBI include five key aspects in their Model of Evidence-based Practice: evidence generation, evidence synthesis, evidence transfer, evidence utilisation and global health. In addition to considering international evidence related to the feasibility, appropriateness, meaningfulness and effectiveness of health care interventions and incorporating this evidence into systematic reviews, JBI globally disseminate information in the form of their *Best Practice Information* summary sheets. They also design programmes to enable the effective implementation of evidence and evaluation of its impact on health care practice.

---

## Box 8.4   Databases

### The Cochrane Database of Systematic Reviews

Systematic reviews undertaken by the Cochrane Collaboration subject to specific evaluation criteria.

### The Database of Abstracts of Reviews of Effects (DARE)

A database maintained and created by the Centre for Reviews and Dissemination at the University of York (CRD): structured abstracts written by CRD reviewers of systematic reviews about the effects of interventions. Inclusion is subject to strict CRD quality criteria.

*(continued)*

*(continued)*

### Cochrane Methodology Register (CMR; Methods Studies)

A bibliography of publications, which report on methods used in the conduct of controlled trials.

### Cochrane Central Register of Controlled Trials

A comprehensive collection of primary research studies.

### The Health Technology Assessment (HTA)

An excellent source of critical reviews.

### NHS Economic Evaluation Database (NHS EED)

A collection of economic evaluations.

---

## Box 8.5    Sources of systematic reviews

Centre for Reviews and Dissemination: www.crd.york.ac.uk/CRDWeb/Home Page.asp
The Cochrane Library: www.thecochranelibrary.com/view/0/index.html
The Campbell Collaboration: www.campbellcollaboration.org/
The Joanna Briggs Institute: joannabriggs.org/

---

## Clinical guidelines

At one time clinical guidelines used to be an area of contention. A quick search of the Internet used to identify many that were not necessarily evidence based. However, a number of established guideline sites now provide access to clear, evidence-based guidance developed according to stringent criteria. Indeed there is even a research programme dedicated to 'reviewing the review' process. The Appraisal of Guidelines Research and Evaluation (AGREE; www.agreetrust.org/), an international collaboration of researchers and policy makers, have developed the AGREE instrument, a systematic framework to enable assessment of key components of guideline quality and to assist in the creation of a coordinated international approach to guideline development.

## Further areas to consider

- How do you ensure you keep your practice up to date and in line with the latest evidence?
- Access some of the websites provided in this chapter and compare the evidence to your current practice.
- Remember to take into account individual patient/client issues when applying evidence – is it the most suitable method for that person?
- Always discuss the evidence with your individual patient, including possible side effects, provide them with the necessary information to enable them to make an informed decision.

<table>
<tr><td>9</td><td></td></tr>
</table>

# Case scenarios

## Overview

This chapter provides both straightforward and more complex case scenarios, for the reader to work through, relating to some of the long-term conditions (LTCs) seen in primary care. Part one considers care management issues for people with a specific LTC. Part two considers care management issues for those with more complex needs. As in earlier chapters, pauses for reflection are provided for each scenario. A suggested course of action is then supplied for each scenario. In practice each person's individual health, cultural and social needs should be taken into consideration when planning care.

## Introduction

The aim of this chapter is to draw together some of the issues that have now been discussed throughout this book and put them into practice through a case study approach. Case scenarios will be provided relating to various conditions, beginning with straightforward cases and progressing to more complex issues. Although based on actual patients all names and identifying details have been anonymised to ensure confidentiality. You are encouraged to read through these and develop an appropriate care plan, based on the information you have read so far and through accessing the relevant evidence-based guideline for the condition being discussed. This can be done as an individual or group learning exercise. Following each scenario suggested courses of action are provided, which are based on appropriate evidence-based guidelines. Remember that in practice each person you see will have individual physical, cultural and social needs, it is impossible to cover all potential scenarios so the ones provided are meant as a guide to assist you in putting theory into practice. Assessment of each person through taking a comprehensive history and carrying out a physical examination (where indicated) will ensure that you determine individual need. This should then be built into a care management plan agreed by both yourself and the person with the LTC that should incorporate education and advice on self-management.

## PART ONE

## Respiratory conditions

### Asthma

The suggested answers to the asthma scenarios are based on information taken from the latest edition of the British Thoracic Society (BTS)/Scottish Intercollegiate Guidelines Network (SIGN) (2014) *Guideline on the Management of Asthma*. For further in-depth information you should access the full version of the guideline, or the guideline currently appropriate for your country.

### *Scenario one*

Bob is a 33-year-old male teacher, who recently had an asthma exacerbation whilst socialising with friends after work. He presented at the Accident and Emergency (A&E) department of his local general hospital, where he was admitted and transferred to the acute medical admissions unit. On admission Bob found it difficult to complete sentences and his peak expiratory flow (PEF) was 40 per cent of predicted (no record was available to hospital staff of his best PEF). His respiratory rate was 27/minute and his heart rate 115/minute. Transfer to the intensive care unit (ICU) for ventilation was discussed, but after instigation of an appropriate treatment plan, his condition stabilised and ventilation was not necessary. He was transferred to a medical ward, from where he was discharged three days later and advised to attend the asthma clinic run in his general practice for treatment review. When reviewing his notes prior to his appointment, the nurse responsible for asthma care in the practice noted that he had not attended for review for over a year, despite two reminder letters. It was also discovered that he had not been collecting his prescriptions for his steroid preventer inhalers for over a year but had been collecting his short acting beta 2 agonist reliever inhalers twice a month.

---

**Pause for reflection**

1. How would you describe Bob's recent asthma exacerbation?
2. What questions do you need to ask him in order to ensure that you take a comprehensive history?
3. Referring to an appropriate evidence-based guideline, e.g. BTS asthma guidelines, develop an appropriate treatment plan for Bob.
4. What general management issues relating to care of patients with asthma are involved in this scenario?
5. How might you prevent future incidences of this type?

## Suggested course of action

1. Bob's asthma exacerbation can be described as acute severe, although in view of the possibility that ventilation was discussed, the hospital notes should be reviewed to determine whether they were concerned at any time that Bob's exacerbation was life-threatening. The presence of features such as exhaustion, confusion, feeble respiratory effort or reduced oxygen saturation (SpO2) levels <92 per cent would have indicated a life-threatening attack. People with a history of a life-threatening attack are known to be at increased risk of mortality.

2. A clear and comprehensive history should be obtained from Bob that should include ascertaining:
   - Whether there have been any changes in Bob's work or home life that has caused his asthma to worsen
   - Why he stopped taking his preventer inhalers
   - Whether he understands the difference between his preventer and reliever inhalers
   - Whether he smokes, or is subject to a smoky atmosphere at home
   - Whether there was any particular reason why he stopped attending asthma review
   - Whether his asthma has prevented him from taking part in his usual activities.

3. Bob's inhaler technique should be reviewed and his PEF rate measured. His best or predicted PEF should be clearly noted. The difference between preventer and reliever therapy should be discussed so Bob is aware of the difference. Any concerns Bob has regarding use of preventer therapy (either financial, or concern re effect of steroids) should be clearly addressed. If any lifestyle changes are identified these should also be discussed along with ways of alleviating or minimising the effects of these. If Bob is smoking, smoking cessation advice should be given. Bob should be encouraged to self-monitor, provided with a peak flow meter and diary and advised what he should do if his PEF measurements reduce. Bob should be advised that effective asthma control means having no day- or night-time symptoms, no exacerbations, no need for rescue medications and no limitations on normal activity with minimal side effects. If Bob finds it difficult to attend the asthma clinic, then alternative arrangements should be discussed. A written self-management plan should be developed that suits Bob's needs, including appropriate review times. As Bob has not been taking his normal preventer inhalers he will need to restart these and then be reviewed at appropriate time intervals to ensure that good control has been achieved and maintained.

4. Despite ordering excessive amounts of reliever therapy and stopping his medication therapy Bob was not reviewed in time to prevent a severe asthma exacerbation. Although Bob had two recall letters no further action was taken.

5. The practice protocol should be reviewed to determine what systems are in place to identify and review people with asthma who are using excessive

cares for her elderly mother. Jennifer struggles with her weight and her BMI is currently 29. Jennifer was started on the biguanide metformin one year ago and her dose has since been increased to 500mg three times daily. She is also taking 75mg aspirin once daily, an angiotensin-converting enzyme (ACE) inhibitor once daily for her blood pressure and a daily statin for her cholesterol. Jennifer doesn't monitor her blood sugars as she finds it stressful to do and upsetting when her readings are raised. Jennifer is attending for her annual review; her blood results, taken prior to the appointment, indicate that her HbA1c is raised at 63.9 mmol/mol and her total cholesterol is 5.5. All other results are within normal limits. Jennifer's blood pressure is raised at 145/90. When discussing her diabetes control Jennifer admits that she frequently forgets her tablets and finds it difficult to stick to a healthy eating regime, often resorting to high calorie, high fat snack or fast food. She has little time for exercise due to the time spent caring for her daughter and mother. She has however stopped taking sugar in her tea. The GP who reviewed her results prior to the review has suggested an increase in both her oral hypoglycaemic and cholesterol medication.

---

### Pause for reflection

1. How can you help Jennifer to improve her diet, lifestyle and concordance with medication?
2. Is increasing her medication a sensible thing to do?
3. What other members of the multi-disciplinary team may be able to help?

---

### Suggested course of action

1. In order to help Jennifer achieve changes in her diet and lifestyle you need to consider what Jennifer wants and how you can empower her to make changes (remember Chapter 5). Emphasising the positives (i.e. congratulating her on stopping taking sugar in her tea) will help encourage Jennifer. Exploring what areas she feels she may be able to change will encourage Jennifer's motivation. For example, although Jennifer finds it difficult to find time to cook, perhaps suggesting she takes her daughter with her when visiting her mother and cooking one healthy meal for all of them may help, rather than cooking for her mother and resorting to fast food for herself. There may be activities that she can do with her daughter that would be beneficial for both of them in increasing her exercise and losing weight. The key is helping her to explore ways in which she feels she can make changes. Discuss the reasons why she doesn't take her medication, does she not like taking tablets or does she forget? A dosset or pill holder box may help; a dosset box is used for storing prescribed medicine and tablets. It is normally a hard plastic grid with sliding clear plastic windows that are labelled with days of the week. A dosset box enables the user to take tablets at regular

intervals. Perhaps a laminated chart on the wall or fridge in her kitchen may act as a useful reminder.

2. In this scenario, as Jennifer readily admits to forgetting her medication, increasing her medication is not a sensible choice. How and when people take their medication and how they feel about it should always be discussed before making any changes. What is important is to emphasise to Jennifer the importance of taking the correct dosages, ascertain what suits her and develop a plan that suits her lifestyle and individual need.

3. Jennifer would probably benefit from a review with a dietitian who will be able to suggest easy ways in which Jennifer can alter her diet that suit her lifestyle (see Chapter 10). Jennifer may also benefit from a referral to social services to see if they can help with caring for her mother and daughter. The local pharmacist may be able to help with organising an easier method to help Jennifer remember her medication. Assistive technology such as text reminders may be a possibility.

This case scenario demonstrates the importance of developing concordance and understanding people's individual needs rather than simply relying on increasing medication.

## Scenario five

Jeff is a 36-year-old married man recently diagnosed with type 2 diabetes. He is not taking any medication at present, but was seen by the dietician within a month of diagnosis. Jeff is a long distance lorry driver and has a young family. He has attended for his first three monthly review, his HbA1c is 74.9 mmol/mol (at diagnosis it was 76 mmol/mol) and his cholesterol is unchanged at 6.5. His blood pressure (BP) remains raised at 150/95 and his BMI is 30. Jeff has a strong family history of both diabetes and cardiovascular disease (CVD), his father had diabetes and died of a myocardial infarction (MI) at age 59 and his 62-year-old mother, who also has diabetes, has poor eyesight and has had two toes amputated. Jeff readily admits that his diet is poor and that when he is not driving he drinks 8–10 pints of beer in the evenings. He feels that developing diabetes was inevitable and that there is little he can do about it.

### Pause for reflection

1. What sort of advice and support can you give Jeff?
2. What pharmacological treatment, if any, would you advise for Jeff?
3. When would be a suitable time for the next review?

1. Jeff is clearly having difficulties coming to terms with the diagnosis and is influenced by his experience of the condition so far. Jeff would benefit from referral to a structured programme of diabetes education that his wife could attend as well. This could be through a locally run scheme such as DESMOND (Diabetes Education and Self Management for Ongoing and Newly Diagnosed Diabetes) if available, or referral to an Expert Patients Programme (EPP). If a suitable programme is not available in your area it is important to develop a structured education programme for Jeff, to ensure that he is fully aware of his condition and potential complications and how these can be avoided with appropriate lifestyle changes. The aim should be to not only improve his knowledge and skills but also to motivate him to effectively self-manage. As with Jennifer, you need to empower and support Jeff to make changes to his diet and lifestyle through exploring how he feels about the diagnosis and what changes he feels he could make. Inviting Jeff to bring his wife to the consultation may also be helpful, as he may have found it difficult to discuss the diagnosis and the potential implication of having diabetes with her. Jeff will need particular support in assisting him in making dietary changes and reducing his alcohol intake on his rest days. Jeff should be asked about any potential problems with his diabetes, such as erectile dysfunction, neuropathy and/or depression, so these can be dealt with appropriately.

2. In view of Jeff's weight metformin would be suitable first line therapy in achieving normoglycaemia, providing his renal function tests are normal. Although Jeff has not altered his lifestyle at this stage it is important to begin the process of glycaemic control. It is imperative that Jeff realises that the medication is to assist him in achieving normoglycaemia and is not a 'quick fix'. Jeff also needs to be prescribed an ACE inhibitor for his BP as his BP has been consistently raised and a statin for his cholesterol, as his cardiovascular risk profile is poor. Jeff should be offered low dose aspirin 75 mg daily as he has significant cardiovascular risk factors (family history, hypertension, features of the metabolic syndrome). How and when to take his medication should be incorporated into a personalised treatment plan.

3. Jeff needs to be seen in a month to assess his BP. A lipid profile and HbA1c should be repeated in three months followed by a review. Jeff should also be supported in the interim to encourage him in making lifestyle changes and this will depend on his individual need.

# Musculoskeletal conditions

## Osteoporosis

The suggested answer to the osteoporosis scenario is based on information taken from the Clinical Knowledge Summaries (CKS 2013a) clinical topic *Osteoporosis*. For further in-depth information you should access the latest evidence-based summary, or the guideline currently appropriate for your country.

## Scenario six

Mrs T is an active 79-year-old woman who has attended for review at her GP surgery, following recent hospitalisation and rehabilitation for a recent fragility hip fracture, which occurred when she had a simple fall at home after getting out of bed. Apart from the fracture Mrs T lives on her own and has little other medical history of note, however her BMI is low at 19. Prior to the fracture she was extremely independent. At the time of consultation she is staying with her daughter but is keen to return home as soon as she is able.

### Pause for reflection

1. What condition may have caused Mrs T's fracture?
2. What other tests may you need to carry out to confirm your diagnosis?
3. What treatment and advice should be offered to Mrs T?

### Suggested course of action

1. Although in general a diagnosis of osteoporosis is made by measuring bone mineral density (BMD), in Mrs T's case she has had a fragility fracture from a standing height and is over 75, so a diagnosis of osteoporosis can be assumed.
2. There is no need for BMD measurement. However differential diagnosis such as skeletal metastases or multiple myeloma should be ruled out, if indicated from the clinical history. If a secondary cause is suspected this should be investigated, for example thyroid function test to exclude hyperthyroidism, bone, liver and renal biochemistry to exclude osteomalacia.
3. Mrs T should be started on a biphosphonate (alendronate or risedronate) and clear verbal and written instructions given on how to take it. If she has a history of any upper gastrointestinal disorder alendronate should not be used. Dietary intake should be discussed and calcium and vitamin D prescribed if dietary intake is inadequate. Mrs T may also benefit from referral to a dietitian to ensure adequate nutritional intake, as she is underweight. She should also be asked if she has had any other falls in the past year and if so the frequency, context and characteristics of the falls. A multifactorial falls risk assessment should be offered if she has had recurrent falls or demonstrates abnormalities of gait or balance. Other lifestyle measures that can help reduce bone thinning should be discussed, these include:

## Scenario ten

Mrs Jones is a 92-year-old woman who has osteoarthritis, COPD, CVD and heart failure. She lives alone and up until recently had been relatively independent. Within the past year she has had a number of falls, which have resulted in numerous hospital admissions. It has been suggested that she moves into a residential care home, Mrs Jones is keen to return to her own home but has agreed that she needs extra support.

### Pause for reflection

1.  What type of care would be the most suitable for Mrs Jones?
2.  What type of skills would the nurse responsible for Mrs Jones's care require?
3.  How can the nurse responsible for her care help maximise the quality of Mrs Jones's care?

### Suggested course of action

1.  Mrs Jones has complex care needs and is at high risk of repeated admission to hospital. She has a number of co-morbidities and will consequently be taking a number of different medications. To enable her to remain at home requires a case management approach to her care to coordinate a health and social care package that meets her specific needs. The principles behind case management include enabling Mrs Jones to have a personalised care plan based on her individual needs and choice and to ensure that appropriate referral is made to the correct agencies and health and social care professionals when it is needed.
2.  In order to provide the care that Mrs Jones requires, the nurse responsible for her case management will require a number of key skills, these include:
    *   Advanced level assessment skills
    *   Supplementary or independent prescribing qualification
    *   Health promotion skills
    *   The ability to coordinate care across agencies
    *   The ability to support self-care and independence
    *   Leadership and management skills.
3.  Once Mrs Jones has been assessed and a care plan developed the nurse responsible for Mrs Jones's case management will need to:
    *   Work in partnership with Mrs Jones's GP and other agencies, such as social services
    *   Work collaboratively with other professionals, carers and relatives
    *   Make regular contact with Mrs Jones
    *   Order investigations where necessary

- Update medical records
- Ensure Mrs Jones is prescribed and receives appropriate medication
- Educate Mrs Jones, her carers and relatives about her condition and how to identify exacerbations
- Liaise with secondary care
- Prepare Mrs Jones and her family for any condition changes and support choices about end of life care when this proves necessary.

## Scenario eleven

Tim is 35, he has epilepsy and learning disabilities and was diagnosed with type 2 diabetes three years ago for which he remains diet controlled. He lives with his mother and sister (his main carer) and attends a centre on a daily basis where he enjoys carpentry and is relatively independent. However he has had one hospital admission in the past year, following hitting his head at the centre after suffering a seizure. His sister is concerned that Tim's weight is creeping up, despite eating healthily at home. His BMI has gone up from 27 to 29 within the past two years. Tim is attending the surgery for an annual review of both his epilepsy and diabetes.

### Pause for reflection

1. What type of care would be most suitable for Tim?
2. What types of issues need to be discussed in Tim's review?
3. What other nurses and health care professionals may be helpful in providing advice to Tim and his family?

### Suggested course of action

1. Tim would be best managed through a disease/care management approach for high risk patients, with a multi-disciplinary team providing high quality evidence-based care to achieve optimum health and reduce risks of complications and deterioration. The nurse conducting Tim's review should ensure that the information from the review is shared between the necessary health care professionals involved in Tim's care, Tim and his carer.
2. Tim's review will need to consider issues related to both his epilepsy and diabetes, including prior measurement of all physical parameters relating to the diabetes review. Regarding his epilepsy Tim and his sister should be asked about seizure control, adverse effects of medication and compliance with medication. As Tim has been admitted during the last year following a seizure it should be ensured that Tim is taking his medication correctly,

or omission of care. Although the case studies are purposefully generic and have not discussed any particular cultural or social issues you should consider the specific needs in your area and incorporate these into your care planning and implementation.

## Key points

- Assess each patient on an individual basis and take into account cultural and social as well as health needs.
- Ensure that you have a method within your practice area to identify people requiring a disease/care management or case management approach.
- Incorporate advice on self-management into individual care plans.

## Further areas to consider

- Where case management schemes are not available who takes responsibility for people with complex care needs?
- How do you ensure that records are shared between appropriate health and social care professionals?
- If you are providing a disease/care management or case management approach how do you ensure that your educational needs are met?

<table>
<tr><td>

10

</td><td>

# Nutritional and medication management

</td></tr>
</table>

---

## Overview

The importance of multi-disciplinary team working was discussed in Chapter 3. This chapter explores the importance of dietary and medicines management in the care of people with a long-term condition (LTC).

**Part one: nutritional management.** The relationship between both obesity and malnutrition and LTCs is explored and practical guidelines are provided relating to assessment and management of a patient's nutritional status, including why weight management advice is important.

**Part two: medication management.** Department of Health (DH) figures indicate that 50 per cent of patients with LTCs fail to take their medicines properly. Schemes that have been shown to be successful in encouraging patients to take their medicines correctly are reviewed along with the importance of team working with pharmacists. This section will also discuss the role of non-medical prescribing in the management of LTCs.

---

## Introduction

This book has so far explored the ways in which nurses working in the primary care environment can support people with LTCs. The importance of team working and appropriate referral has been discussed and the need for a multi-disciplinary coordinated and systematic approach to care. The aim of this chapter is to discuss two particularly important aspects of LTC care, nutrition and medicines management. Part one of this chapter, written by a registered dietitian, reviews the relationship between nutritional status and LTCs focusing on aetiology, associated health risks and management of both over-nutrition (obesity) and under-nutrition (malnutrition). Part two reviews the importance of medicine management, the importance of the role of the pharmacist in educating and supporting people with LTCs and the impact of non-medical prescribing on the management of people with LTCs.

## PART ONE[1]

# Nutritional management of patients with LTCs

Poor nutrition can be both the cause and cause of concern in many patients living with an LTC. Successful dietary intervention can reduce the risk of further complications and improve quality of life. All health care professionals working in primary care should be able to identify patients in need of dietary evaluation and have an obligation to include other members of the multi-disciplinary team within each individual care plan, to offer appropriate dietary advice and support. A dietitian or dietetic team may be involved or consulted in the care of these patients in order to assist them to address and achieve their nutritional needs.

Malnutrition directly translates to 'bad nutrition'. It is a term used to describe both over-nutrition i.e. overweight and under-nutrition i.e. underweight. Sometimes patients tend to follow a trend according to their condition e.g. type 2 diabetes is strongly associated with the over-nourished patient. Other times patients present very differently e.g. a chronic pulmonary obstructive disease (COPD) patient may be under- or overweight and both states have direct influence on how that patient's condition should be managed. This section is going to focus on both sides of this axis and how they will influence the patient with LTCs.

## Obesity – 'over-nutrition'

The incidence of obesity, in the UK and worldwide, is increasing rapidly with no sign of slowing down. In 1993 13 per cent of men and 16 per cent of women were obese but in 2012 this had risen to 24 per cent for men and 25 per cent for women. Further to this the number of adults classed as overweight increased from 57 per cent to 66 per cent in men and from 49 per cent to 57 per cent in women (Health and Social Care Information Centre 2014). Worryingly rates of childhood obesity are also rising, having potential consequences for future patients and the health as a nation. Obesity is strongly associated with other medical problems, notably the chronic LTCs highlighted in this book (Table 10.1). In addition excess weight can have significant implications for self-esteem and mental health influencing motivation and potentially someone's drive for long-term self-care. In 2013 the DH stated that health problems associated with being overweight or obese cost the NHS more than £5 billion every year. It is estimated that by 2050 this will increase to £50 billion (National Obesity Forum 2014).

It is vital the patient understands that 'overweight' and 'obesity' are clinical terms with health implications rather than just a question or judgement of how someone looks (National Institute for Health and Care Excellence (NICE) 2006a). Having an honest and open conversation with patients about their weight is likely to be the first step towards supporting dietary changes.

---

Pause for reflection

---

What impact has obesity had on the incidence of LTCs in your area?

**Table 10.1 Health risks of obesity**

| Greatly increased risk | Moderately increased risk | Slightly increased risk |
| --- | --- | --- |
| Type 2 diabetes | Cardiovascular | Certain cancers, including colon, kidney, |
| Gallbladder disease | diseases | prostate (men), post-menopausal breast |
| Dyslipidaemia | Hypertension | and endometrial (women) |
| Insulin resistance | Osteoarthritis (knee) | Reproductive hormone abnormalities |
| Breathlessness | Hyperuricaemia and | Polycystic Ovary Syndrome |
| Sleep apnoea | gout | Impaired fertility |
| | | Lower back pain |
| | | Increases anaesthetic risk |
| | | Foetal defects associated with maternal obesity |

Source: World Health Organisation (WHO) (1998)

## Classification of obesity

Body mass index (BMI) is a widely used and recognised measurement of weight for height in adults. It is defined as weight in kilograms divided by height in metres squared (kg/m$^2$). From this worldwide classifications of obesity can be determined (Table 10.2). However, results should be interpreted with an element of a 'rough guide' as BMI does not take into account body composition i.e. muscle vs fat. In a clinical setting using basic anthropometry such as waist circumference can be a successful alternative classification system and a way to monitor patient progress away from the weighing scales. A high proportion of abdominal fat is related to an increased health risk, notably of type 2 diabetes and cardiovascular disease (Table 10.3).

As BMIs are increasing on a global scale it is easier for people to dismiss BMIs of 25–30 or slightly higher waist circumferences as 'normal'. Once a measurement is taken the long-term health risks should be explained (NICE 2006a). The patient needs

**Table 10.2 Classification of overweight and obesity**

| Classification | BMI (kg/m$^2$) |
| --- | --- |
| Healthy weight | 18.5–24.9 |
| Overweight | 25–29.9 |
| Obesity I | 30–34.9 |
| Obesity II | 35–39.9 |
| Obesity III | 40 or more |

Table 10.3  Waist circumference and risk factors

|  | *Increased risk* | *Substantial risk* |
|---|---|---|
| Men | ≥94cm (~37 inches) | ≥102cm (~40 inches) |
| Women | ≥80cm (~32 inches) | ≥88cm (~35 inches) |

Source: adapted from WHO (1998)

to recognise how their current weight will influence health outcomes and it is easy for an overweight patient to become increasingly overweight, particularly if activity levels are reducing secondary to a physical decline or older age.

## *Aetiology of obesity*

In theory weight gain is a simple consequence of an imbalance of energy input to energy output (i.e. positive energy balance). It is generally considered to be the result of energy-rich, nutrient-poor diets coupled with sedentary lifestyle. In reality there are many influencing factors on this equation and all aspects of a patient's diet and lifestyle, including any LTC, should be considered in order to make appropriate and realistic interventions.

Genetic influence on obesity is widely discussed and some research has shown familial characteristics between overweight parents and their children. People will exhibit a body type or 'somatotype' often similar to family members. For example endomorphic individuals generally present as 'short and round' with an easier predisposition to carry body fat, whereas an ectomorphic individual will generally be 'tall and long' and find it difficult to gain weight. There is also a lot of 'grey area' here where the body will be a mix of various somatotypes and often 'shapes' such as apple or pear are used to describe the overall fat distribution on the body. The importance of this is that patients should be discouraged from comparing themselves to others who may not be struggling with their weight or apply a 'one size fits all' approach to weight management strategies.

It is overwhelmingly evident that obesity is not just the result of genetic influence but also of environmental, social and psychological influences. With appropriate interventions even subjects with genetic predispositions should be able to maintain their weight within a normal range (Barasi 2003).

Pause for reflection

What environmental, psychological and social influences impact on the development of obesity?

## Management of obesity

Obesity can be managed in primary care by a motivated, well-informed multi-disciplinary team. Recognition and identification of the treatment groups that require further advice and support is the vital first step (Table 10.4).

**Table 10.4 Treatment groups**

---

Treatment or advice should be offered to:
- Patients with a BMI of 30 or above
- Patients with a BMI of 28 and above with co-morbidities e.g. coronary heart disease (CHD), diabetes
- Patients with any degree of overweight coinciding with diabetes, other severe risk factors or serious disease
- Patients who self-refer, where appropriate

Special consideration should be given to:
- Parents of families with more than one overweight or obese member

Preventative advice should be offered to high risk individuals:
- Patients with a family history of obesity
- Smokers
- Patients with learning difficulties
- Low-income groups

---

Source: adapted from National Obesity Forum (2008)

As well as initial assessment of classification of obesity (as previously discussed) collecting information about weight history including past history of dieting is important. This can then be used to stimulate conversation about readiness for change, barriers to change and also current diet and activity levels. The key with all patients is to find their motivation to change dietary habits and lose weight. While the patient may appear motivated to change they may be looking for a 'quick fix' or feel they want to be told what to do. Ultimately the multi-disciplinary team can advise on how weight loss can be achieved and barriers overcome but the patient has to maintain the changes that are likely to be involved when adjusting long-standing habits or behaviours. Therefore finding their motivation to do so will be vital in helping them to change (see Chapter 5). Explaining the health risks of obesity may be influential but other factors may take priority in a patient's mind such as being able to play with children or grandchildren or fitting into a favourite pair of jeans or dress. Whatever the motivating factor it should be taken into account and re-visited with patients to keep dietary changes on track.

There are several treatment options for obesity, but all are underpinned with achieving a negative energy balance with healthy eating advice and promotion of exercise. Although the message appears to be simple and not as glamorous as the latest 'fad' or 'celebrity' diet it is the only way to achieve sustainable lifestyle changes. Diets with grand claims or promises of substantial weight loss, in often very limited time periods, should be discouraged. These diets are usually based upon restrictive eating patterns and poor nutritional quality and can be particularly damaging for LTCs, for example a low carbohydrate diet is unsuitable for the patient with diabetes. A calorie deficit based on a balanced diet is easily achieved with a little thought and planning. Similarly over the counter slimming aids are becoming increasingly popular usually based on 'natural' components which seem appealing despite their often expensive cost. Unfortunately most of the success found with these products is secondary to placebo rather than any miracle ingredient. Guiding your patient through the minefield of the commercial weight loss industry can be challenging.

Other interventions for weight loss such as medications and surgery should only be considered after three to six months of the first line treatments (i.e. diet and lifestyle changes). Interestingly while a patient may feel these options are the answer to their weight loss they have to lose weight first and continue to maintain dietary changes even with drug therapy or surgical intervention. Guidelines on who is appropriate for second line treatments are outlined in Table 10.5.

Table 10.5  A guide to deciding level of intervention

| BMI classification | Waist circumference | | | Co-morbidities present |
|---|---|---|---|---|
| | Low | High | Very high | |
| Overweight | | | | |
| Obesity I | | | | |
| Obesity II | | | | |
| **Obesity III** | | | | |

☐ General advice on healthy weight and lifestyle
▨ Diet and physical activity
▩ Diet and physical activity; consider drugs
■ Diet and physical activity; consider surgery

Source: adapted from NICE (2006a)

Multicomponent interventions should be put in place to encourage sustainable lifestyle change with a consistent message coming from all members of the primary care team. Look for lifestyle groups, exercise on prescription schemes and healthy eating initiatives such as fruit and vegetable boxes in your area that may be of benefit to your patient. Treatment options should remain patient-centred and consider what the individual will respond best to. For example while a group setting may suit one person, someone else may feel overwhelmed with this and as such the intervention will fail and as a result the patient will also feel they have failed, thus perpetuating the cycle of potential previous failures to lose weight in the past. Dietetic resources are often limited and therefore dietitians will rely on other members of the primary care team to reiterate healthy eating messages and point patients in the right direction either with or without initial dietetic consultation. Quite often it can be more beneficial for a patient to take advice from a team member they have gained trust and respect for, for example an LTC specialist nurse. In addition talking about weight openly and honestly during a non-weight focused consultation may be the best way to capture a patient's motivation and stimulate a positive conversation about changes that could be made.

### Pause for reflection

Do you know what schemes are available in your area? If so how do you ensure you inform your patients/clients?

## Targets of treatment

Achievable, realistic weight loss goals should be set with the patient. It is recognised that a 5–10 per cent loss of original weight can bring about substantial benefits to health (Table 10.6). A maximum loss of 0.5–1kg per week is ideal. This can be achieved by maintaining a deficit of 400–600kcal per day. In real terms this could be the result of changing a high kcal snack to a portion of fruit and reducing a portion of starchy carbohydrates with the main meal for example. Remember that the kcal deficit should aim to be from elements of the diet that do not lead to nutritional inadequacies, such as cutting out whole food groups. The Eatwell Plate is a helpful tool in consideration for reasonable changes and can help focus a patient on what should be in the diet as well as what they think they can reduce.

**Table 10.6 Benefits of a 10kg weight loss in a 100kg individual i.e. 10% weight loss**

| Indication | Improvement to health |
| --- | --- |
| Mortality | >20% ↓ total mortality<br>>30% ↓ diabetes related deaths<br>>40% ↓ obesity related cancers |
| Blood pressure | 10mmHg ↓ systolic<br>20mmHg ↓ diastolic |
| Lipids | 10% total cholesterol<br>15% ↓ LDL<br>30% ↓ triglycerides<br>8% ↑ HDL |
| Diabetes | 30–50% ↓ fasting glucose<br>50% ↓ risk of diabetes developing<br>15% ↓ in HbA1c |
| Physical complications | Improved back and joint pain<br>Improved lung function<br>Reduced frequency of sleep apnoea |

Source: adapted from Jung (1997)

Other examples of practical lifestyle changes are listed below. Small goals like this are easier to set and therefore easier to maintain. Discouraging patients to try to change 'everything' will help them to focus their efforts on areas of their diet and lifestyle that will make the biggest influence. Weight loss should be ideally within three months of making changes and maintained for 12 months as an indicator of success (NICE 2006a). Reaching a 'plateau' with weight loss is normal. As the body becomes accustomed to less food and/or more exercise weight will be harder to lose. At this point further diet or lifestyle changes will need to be put into place and again discussing motivation and readiness for change with the patient will be beneficial to ensure they stay focused to achieve their target goals.

Examples of diet or lifestyle changes to consider with patients include:

- Avoid skipping breakfast. Choose a balanced option such as plain cereal with semi-skimmed milk and a glass of fresh orange juice.
- Swap biscuit snacks mid morning with a handful of dried fruits.
- Reduce the number of spoons of pasta/rice/potatoes with main meal; but add in two extra spoons of vegetables.
- Choose to eat main meal on a smaller plate to help control serving sizes.
- Try to have a low kcal yoghurt instead of a cream based pudding.
- Go for a walk or cycle in the evening to provide some distraction and avoid extra snacks being eaten in front of the TV.
- To walk up and down the stairs 'x' number of times during the day for additional exercise.

## Key resources

- NICE (2006a) Clinical Guideline 42: *Obesity*
- International Obesity Task Force: www.iotf.org
- British Dietetic Association (BDA) Weight Wise Campaign: www.bdaweight wise.com
- Food Standards Agency (FSA) website: www.food.gov.uk
- Eatwell Plate: *Your Guide to Eatwell Plate, Helping You Eat a Healthier Diet* (2014): www.gov.uk/government

## Key points

- Obesity rates in the UK are increasing for both adults and children.
- Obesity is a serious health risk with strong links with many chronic diseases.
- The level of obesity and associated health risks can be determined by BMI and waist circumference.
- Gradual, realistic weight loss goals should be set with the patient to achieve sustainable lifestyle changes.
- Dietary modification and exercise promotion are the basis of weight management.
- Medications and surgery may be suitable for some patients.
- 10 per cent weight loss can bring about substantial improvements to health.

## Malnutrition – 'under-nutrition'

In the clinical setting the underweight patient is more commonly referred to as the malnourished patient or a patient at risk of malnutrition. A patient that is underweight is going to present with a different set of health problems that will influence how well an LTC is managed or treated. The estimated number of malnourished individuals in the UK is worrying. It is estimated that there are in excess of 3 million people in the

**Table 10.7 Physiological and psychological consequences of malnutrition**

| Effect | Consequence |
| --- | --- |
| Impaired immune response | Impaired ability to fight infection |
| Reduced muscle strength and fatigue | Inactivity and reduced ability to work, shop, cook and self-care. Poor muscle function may result in falls, and in the case of poor respiratory muscle function result in poor cough pressure – delaying expectoration and recovery from chest infection |
| Inactivity | In bed-bound patients, this may result in pressure ulcers and venous blood clots, which can break loose and embolise |
| Loss of temperature regulation | Hypothermia with consequent further loss of muscle strength |
| Impaired wound healing | Increased wound-related complications, such as infections and un-united fractures |
| Impaired ability to regulate salt and fluid | Predisposes to over-hydration, or dehydration |
| Impaired ability to regulate periods | Impaired reproductive function |
| Impaired foetal and infant programming | Malnutrition during pregnancy predisposes to common chronic diseases, such as cardiovascular disease, stroke and diabetes (in adulthood) |
| Specific nutrient deficiencies | Anaemia and other consequences of iron, vitamin and trace element deficiency |
| Impaired psycho-social function | Even when uncomplicated by disease, malnutrition causes apathy, depression, introversion, self-neglect, hypochondriasis, loss of libido and deterioration in social interactions (including mother-child bonding) |
| Additional effects on children and adolescents | Growth failure and stunting, delayed sexual development, reduced muscle mass and strength, impaired neuro-cognitive development, rickets and increased lifetime osteoporosis risk |

Source: Elia and Russell (2009)

UK affected by malnutrition and 93 per cent of those reside in the community and therefore under the care of primary care teams (British Association for Parenteral and Enteral Nutrition (BAPEN) 2014). It is recognised that these patients have higher use of health care services, more medications, more hospital admissions, longer hospital stays, increased risk of infections, poor wound healing, poorer health outcomes and higher rates of mortality. It is estimated that the cost to the NHS is in excess of £13 billion per year, over double the estimated cost for obesity (Elia and Russell 2009). Malnutrition affects every system of the body and has serious consequences for the management of LTCs. An overview of malnutrition consequences is described in Table 10.7.

## Classification of malnutrition

As with obesity the BMI can be a rough guide to indicate someone's risk of malnutrition. In addition previous *unintentional* weight loss should also be considered. In the UK the most recognised and validated screening tool for malnutrition is Malnutrition Universal Screening Tool (MUST). It provides a scoring system to identify not just those at risk but also the level of risk (low, medium, high) and therefore supports the application of appropriate care plans for those patients (NICE 2006b).

MUST considers current BMI and notes that a BMI <18.5 is high risk, 18.5–20 is medium risk and >20 is low risk. However it also adds the addition of previous unintentional weight loss which can have a strong influence on overall score. Weight loss over the past 3–6 months should be considered i.e. short-term loss not long-term gradual losses. If the loss is greater than 10 per cent of body weight a high risk score is applied. Between 5 and 10 per cent is medium risk and <5 per cent is low risk. The reason this is so important is that someone with a relatively normal or even high BMI can still be at risk of malnutrition when a significant amount of weight has been lost over a short period of time. MUST allows that patient to be identified and care plans put into place before the patient needs to lose considerable amounts of weight to have a low BMI and potentially be at higher risk of poor health outcomes before interventions are taken. The final score of MUST is applying an acute disease effect score, that is whether the patient is acutely unwell and because of that they have eaten little or no food for 5 days or more. While a patient may be eating less than normal this score requires professional judgement as to whether it accounts for a significant score. It is important to remember this should be applied to an acute illness therefore chronic conditions with reduced food intake over some time does not warrant this score to be added. Finally the scores are added together to produce an overall risk score which involves a score of 0 a low risk, score of 1 a medium risk and a score of 2 or more a high risk. Guidance on how to complete MUST scores can be provided by your local dietetic department or by looking online at BAPEN.org.uk.

## *Aetiology of malnutrition*

Again the theory here is simple. An imbalance of energy but this time there is more energy expended than is taken in and unintentional weight loss is the result. Usually the resultant weight loss is not taken from the body's fat stores but initially muscle mass as it is an easier source of calories for the body to utilise, albeit with less efficiency. Patients will often complain of 'lack of strength' and lethargy often coupled with a reduction in physical ability as a result. They will also often present with a similar physical appearance of a 'gaunt' face, loss of muscle tone and protruding bones (often on the upper body). Vulnerable population groups are those with chronic diseases, elderly people, those recently discharged from hospital and those who are poor or socially isolated (BAPEN 2003). Malnutrition is often under-recognised and under-treated in the community.

Reduced appetite is probably the most common cause for poor dietary intake and malnutrition. The appetite of an individual is not only affected by physical health but also mental and social influences. Losing the desire for food can often be a telling sign that someone is unwell and can leave the patient feeling very different to their 'normal' self. It is widely understood that as individuals get older their appetite may decrease, but this does not necessarily mean that weight loss is inevitable. As people age it is felt their activity levels also reduce in line with this and as such energy balance can be maintained. Appetite is sensitive to psychological well-being and whether changes to physical health, social situation or mental health have influenced appetite, addressing these reasons will be necessary to help the patient understand how their current intake is a result and needs to be changed. A summary of influences to nutritional intake is described in Table 10.8. It is important to remember that the influences are often interrelated. For example someone with dysphagia may also suffer with low mood due to the resultant advice to change diet to a soft or pureed texture which they may be self-conscious or upset about.

**Table 10.8  A summary of influences to nutritional intake**

| | |
|---|---|
| Medical conditions | • Persistent pain or nausea (such as in cancer)<br>• Mental health conditions such as depression<br>• Swallowing difficulties (dysphagia)<br>• Persistent diarrhoea or vomiting<br>• Constipation |
| Physical factors | • Lack of dentition or poor oral health, including ill-fitting dentures<br>• Loss of smell or taste sensation (possibly due to medication or ageing)<br>• Physical disability influencing ability to prepare/cook meals |
| Social factors | • Living alone and social isolation<br>• Limited knowledge (regarding nutrition and/or cooking)<br>• Low income or poverty<br>• Reduced mobility<br>• Drug or alcohol dependence |

On the other side of the balance increased energy expenditure can be the result of a disease state; however it is more likely because of the consequences of that disease. For example poor respiratory function in COPD means the patient needs more calories (energy) to support difficulties in breathing. Independent risk factors for malnutrition may also include reduced absorption of macro and/or micro nutrients, for example following abdominal surgical procedures or increased losses or altered requirements secondary to enterocutaneous fistula or burns.

## Management of malnutrition

Increasing energy intake is key in treating malnutrition. First line dietary advice can be offered by any member of a multi-disciplinary team and simple steps can be suggested to try to improve overall nutritional intake. Using a food first approach is vital in putting in appropriate care plans for these patients. Practical advice includes trying to eat 'little and often' during the day, choosing higher calorie and protein options, fortifying foods with additional high calorie and protein foods or trying to include nourishing drinks in between meals. Other aspects of eating also need to be considered such as: would the patient benefit from carers to support meal preparation, would a meal delivery service be helpful or does the patient need supportive aids for eating (such as adapted cutlery or high sided plates)? In addition, a little activity may be beneficial to the patient to stimulate appetite if it is possible for the patient to do so.

Patients with LTCs may feel a high calorie diet contradicts previous healthy eating advice they may have been given. Encouraging them to maintain a balanced diet (as per the Eatwell Plate) is important to remember as well as offering reassurance that the diet can be used as a short-term measure and/or it would be a priority to prevent further weight loss or promote weight gain.

Further treatment options may include the use of oral nutritional supplements (ONS), however their use should be considered carefully. It is well documented that these products, more often presented in a drink form, are poorly prescribed and managed and can lead to costly waste for the NHS (Elia et al. 2005). Ultimately the use of supplements should only be considered if patients meet the Advisory Committee for Borderline Substances (ACBS) prescribing criteria and have been identified through MUST screening or according to NICE criteria to be at nutritional risk.

The aim of ONS is to provide additional nutrition to support the patient's food intake (typically an additional 250–600kcal/day). When used appropriately they can lead to improved patient outcomes (Stratton et al. 2003). Where they should not be used is to provide sole nutrition for a patient by replacing meals. In addition if the extra nutrition can be provided by normal foods and drinks this should be preferable as often this is more successful and palatable for the patient. Often regional NHS Trusts will provide guidelines (produced by Medicines Management and/or Dietetic Teams) as to which patients are appropriate for ONS and also prescribing guidelines with first line ONS choices.

There may be situations whereby a patient at risk of malnutrition with an LTC may require further nutrition support in the form of artificial feeding such as nasogastric

(NG) or percutaneous endoscopic gastrostomy (PEG). Careful consideration should be given to whether this is appropriate for the patient and the multi-disciplinary team discussions with the patient are key to decide if this is a justifiable option.

## Targets of treatment

In order to monitor malnutrition interventions MUST screening is recommended to be completed monthly in the community to assess patient progression. More often the aim of treatment will be to promote weight gain. However, there may be situations where prevention of further weight loss is felt to be a more appropriate treatment aim. Improvements to appetite can be monitored via the use of a food chart/diary and by asking the patient their feelings towards food. A summary of a patient's nutritional care plan is described in Table 10.9.

### Table 10.9 Nutritional care plan

A patient's nutritional care plan should:

- set aims and objectives of treatment
- treat any underlying conditions
- include treatment of the malnutrition with food and/or ONS where appropriate. Patients who are unable to meet their nutritional requirements orally may require artificial nutritional support, e.g. enteral or parenteral nutrition. None of these methods is exclusive and combinations of any or all may be needed. If subjects are overweight or obese, follow local guidelines for weight management
- reassess subjects identified at nutritional risk as they move through care settings

Source: adapted from BAPEN (2011)

## Key resources

- NICE (2006b) Clinical Guideline 32: *Nutrition Support in Adults*
- BAPEN website: www.bapen.org.uk
- Malnutrition Pathway website: www.malnutritionpathway.co.uk

## Key points

- The estimated number of malnourished adults in the UK is worryingly high.
- There are numerous clinical consequences associated with the malnourished patient that could affect the successful management of LTCs.

## NPC Community Pharmacy Framework Collaborative (CPFC)

The CPFC was another national initiative supported by the DH and hosted by the MMS team based at the NPC in Liverpool (NPC 2007). Collaborative methodology was used, as previously, to achieve sustainable quality improvement in medicines management for the 28 teams involved (host PCTs in each of the strategic health authorities (SHAs) in England). Project facilitators were recruited by the host PCTs to support the work. The overall goal was stated as: 'To realise the benefits of increasing the range and quality of services provided from community pharmacies as an integral part of the NHS'.

Aims included:

- Promoting public health and encourage self-care through community pharmacies
- To improve health by assessing and attending to the pharmaceutical needs of local people and individual patients
- Increasing patient choice, access and convenience and improving the patient experience
- To develop clinically effective and cost effective pharmaceutical services that build on the strengths of community pharmacy teams working within a multidisciplinary environment
- Expanding primary care through commissioning of new medicines management and pharmaceutical services.

(NPC 2007)

The specific objectives set to contribute to these aims included to:

- Increase patient choice
- Increase interventions in LTCs
- Reduce medicine related problems
- Increase public health interventions
- Increase locally commissioned services
- Decrease waste by using interventions
- Decrease the burden on GPs by using interventions.

(NPC 2007)

Programme measures were collected at two levels each month, within individual pharmacies and within the host organisation, to measure improvement activity. There were six pharmacy measures and five spread measures overall (although some measures had more than one part). Full details of all the measures and noteworthy examples from the areas involved can be accessed from the final report (NPC 2007). Examples included: *Pharmacy measure 4: Number of face-to-face medicines use reviews (MURs) completed per head of PCT population (increase is an improvement)*.

The number of MURs, which is part of the advanced level of the community pharmacy contract, increased rapidly and then levelled out. Examples of individual improvements provided in the report included one pharmacy increasing from zero

MURs per week to 6.25 MURs per week. Systems put into place by various PCTs to support the pharmacies to achieve these targets included:

- Increasing the number of pharmacists accredited to conduct MURs
- Increasing the number of accredited consultation rooms.

In addition, community pharmacists were advised to:

- Focus on uncomplicated patients suitable for an MUR
- Keep the duration of an MUR session to a reasonable time (no more than 15 minutes)
- Increase pharmacists' confidence with tips on interview techniques, body language and taking a positive approach
- Communicate with GP practices to explain the MUR process and paperwork
- Explain action GPs should take in response to recommendations on MUR forms
- Identify key person and establish a communication process in both GP practice and pharmacy
- Highlight the importance for pharmacists to actively get involved with MURs.

Pharmacy measures 4a and 4b were particularly relevant to people with LTCs.

*4a. The percentage of MURs completed for a long-term condition agreed with the PCT (increase is an improvement).*
*4b. The percentage that reduce medicines waste (increase is an improvement).*

As with pharmacy measure 4, MURs increased rapidly, then levelled out. Notable examples included one PCT who used diabetes as their LTC and focused on calibration of glucose meters and people who had more than one meter. Through linking in with Diabetes Week they launched the service across all locality pharmacies, aiding the education programme of encouraging patients to have their meters calibrated annually and raising patients' awareness of the importance of self-care. Pharmacies collected data over a four-week period around patients' current testing, meter usage, meter types and numbers of testing strips being prescribed. The intention was to use this data to provide useful resource material for service development, further patient education programmes and aid in identifying the best way forward to reduce the number of different meters, fluids and glucose strips prescribed.

A number of better practice outcomes related to the CPFC initiative as a whole were noted. In relation to LTCs one PCT who had a high incidence of respiratory disease developed a leaflet to be used as a counselling tool for community pharmacists when dispensing inhalers for patients, particularly those under 16, with asthma and during MURs. This information could then be taken home with them as a resource. The leaflet entitled 'Top Tips for Asthma' was piloted, users liked it but felt stigmatised by the reference to asthma. The leaflet was redeveloped as 'Inhalers . . . Top Tips for users'. Following further patient evaluation and a 100 per cent positive response from patients who found the leaflet useful and felt that it gave them a better understanding of their inhalers, the leaflet was shared with all community pharmacies and other health care professionals.

This summary has just provided a bird's eye view of the good work and innovative projects that have been developed and supported through the initiative. For further details I strongly recommend you access the full report: *Community Pharmacy Framework Collaborative Final Report* (NPC 2007).

## Pause for reflection

What community pharmacy initiatives are you aware of in your area?

A key aim of the NPC collaborative programmes is to share good ideas, rather than continually reinventing the wheel, what initiatives could you adopt in your area?

## NPC Plus Medicines Partnership Programme

The Medicines Partnership Programme was an initiative aimed at enabling patients to get the most out of their medicines through involving them as partners in decision-making about treatment and supporting them in medicine taking. In order to achieve this a process of concordance was used (see also Chapter 4). The NPC describe concordance as 'a process of prescribing and medicine taking based on partnership', although as has been seen earlier in this book concordance has now been expanded to include all aspects of shared decision-making between health care professionals and their patients/clients. Compliance measures patient behaviour, the extent to which a patient takes medicine according to the prescribed instructions, whereas concordance measures a two way process, involving shared decision-making based on partnership which values patients' expertise and beliefs (NPC Plus 2007). In relation to medicine taking NPC Plus (2007) notes that there are a number of reasons why people do not take their medicines, which include:

- Practical difficulties, such as getting to a pharmacy, opening containers and remembering to take medicines
- Lack of information about their condition and the importance of treatment
- Problems with side effects
- Interference with their daily lives
- Beliefs about the medicine, or medicines in general – for example that medicines are unnatural, harmful, addictive, or that they wear off over time.

NPC Plus (2007) suggests that although practical and logistical difficulties may play a part in unintentional non-compliance with medication, most non-compliance is intentional and based on a conscious decision. This includes peoples' beliefs about their medication, how they should be used and how medicine taking fits within their daily lives. Furthermore these beliefs are shaped by a number of factors including culture, education, social circumstances, fears and anxiety, and experience of family and friends. They may misunderstand the nature of their illness and/or treatment or be unsure whether the benefits of taking the treatment outweigh the risks (NPC Plus 2007).

---

If you have ever been prescribed medication did you take it exactly as prescribed, were potential side effects explained to you and/or the potential consequences of not taking the medication as prescribed?

What reasons have patients given to you for not wishing to take their medication, how did you deal with the situation, were you didactic or supportive in achieving mutual agreement?

---

In order to achieve successful concordance NPC Plus has developed a competency framework which includes eight competencies grouped into three key areas, outlined below:

- **Building a partnership**: Patients have enough knowledge to participate as partners and health professionals are prepared for partnership
- **Managing a shared consultation**: Prescribing consultations involve patients as partners
- **Sharing a decision**: Patients are supported in taking medicines.

Development of competencies through a competency framework helps individuals to improve their performance and to do their jobs more effectively. The NPC Plus competency framework, accessible from the report *A Competency Framework for Shared Decision-making with Patients: Achieving Concordance for Taking Medicines* can be used as a starting point for discussion of competencies either by individuals or as a group learning approach. It can help individuals and organisations identify the skills they require, including training and development needs and inform commissioning, development and provision of educational training programmes (NPC Plus 2007).

---

Have you ever used a competency framework, either individually or as a team?

Using the NPC Plus competency framework review your learning needs related to developing concordance.

---

how they would behave until they are placed in the same situation. Appreciate social and cultural influences on people's lives and always treat people as individuals. If you take one message from this book I hope it is that of shared decision-making and concordance and appreciating that those who live with an LTC will have far more knowledge about the impact of the condition on their life than any health care professional can truly appreciate. However it is up to you to share your knowledge with your patients/clients and provide them with the appropriate information with which to make their own decisions. Hopefully the chapter on evidence-based practice will have improved your ability to access knowledge based on up-to-date evidence and ensure that your practice is not based on 'unsubstantiated certainty'. This book has been about sharing knowledge and would not have been written without utilising the excellent sources of information included in the extensive reference list. Hopefully you are now aware of sources that you can add to your 'favourites' list.

Finally remember that you are not alone, in health care we work as part of a team. Respect the knowledge of others, including your patients, their families and carers and above all respect their wishes, the decision regarding their care is ultimately theirs and theirs alone, we can but advise and support them in the decisions that they make.

# References

Acheson, P. (1998) *Independent Inquiry into Inequalities in Health, The Acheson Report.* London: The Stationery Office.

Amrhein, P. C., Miller, W. R., Yahne, C. E., Palmer, M. and Fulcher, L. (2003) Client commitment language during motivational interviewing predicts drug use outcomes. *Journal of Consulting and Clinical Psychology,* 71, 862–878.

An Roinn Slainte Department of Health (2012) *Health in Ireland Key Trends 2012.* Available from: www.dohc.ie/publications/pdf/KeyTrends_2012.pdf?direct=1 (accessed November 2014).

Arthritis Australia (2014) *What Is Arthritis?* Available from: www.arthritisaustralia.com.au/index.php/arthritis-information.html (accessed July 2014).

Arthritis Care (2008) *Ways to Self-Manage.* Available from: www.arthritiscare.org.uk/LivingwithArthritis/Self-management/Waystoself-manage (accessed November 2014).

Arthritis Research UK (2013) *Arthritis Information.* Available from www.arthritisresearchuk.org/arthritis-information/conditions/arthritis.aspx (accessed July 2014).

Asthma UK (2014) *Knowledge Bank.* Available from: www.asthma.org.uk/knowledge-bank-living-with-asthma (accessed December 2014).

Asthma UK Cymru (2008) *A Quarter of a Million Voices . . . and Counting.* Available from: www.asthma.org.uk/news_media/news/a_quarter_feel_hopel.html (accessed July 2008).

Australian Commission on Safety and Quality in Health Care (2014) *Shared Decision Making.* Available from: www.safetyandquality.gov.au/our-work/shared-decision-making/ (accessed November 2014).

Australian Government Department of Health (2012) *Chronic Disease.* Available from: www.health.gov.au/internet/main/publishing.nsf/Content/chronic (accessed June 2014).

Australian Institute of Health and Welfare (AIHW) (2013) *Chronic Diseases.* Available from: www.aihw.gov.au/chronic-diseases/ (accessed November 2014).

Bandura, A. (1977) Self-efficacy: toward a unifying theory of behavioral change. *Psychological Review,* 84, 191–215.

Bandura A. (1995) *Self-efficacy in Changing Societies.* Cambridge: Cambridge University Press.

Barasi, M. (2003) *Human Nutrition: A Health Perspective,* 2nd edn. UK: Arnold Publishers.

Barlow, J., Wright, C., Sheasby, J., Turner, A. and Hainsworth, J. (2002) Self-management approaches for people with chronic conditions: a review. *Patient Education and Counselling,* 48, 177–187.

Barron, S., Balanda, K.P. and Fahy, L. (2010) *Making Chronic Conditions Count: Hypertension, Stroke, Coronary Heart Disease, Diabetes. A systematic approach to estimating and forecasting population prevalence on the island of Ireland. Technical Supplement.* Dublin: Institute of Public Health in Ireland.

Bem, D. J. (1972) Self-perception theory. In Berkowitz, L. (ed.) *Advances in Experimental Social Psychology.* New York: Academic Press.

Bent, N., Tennant, A., Swift, T., Posnett, J., Scuffham, P. and Chamberlain, M. A. (2000) Team approach versus ad-hoc health services for young people with physical disabilities: a retrospective cohort study. *Lancet,* 360, 1280–1286.

Berry, D. (2007) *Healthcare Communication: Theory and Practice.* Maidenhead: Open University Press.

Bernabei, E., Landi, F. and Gamgassi, G. (1998) Randomised trial of impact model of integrated care and case management for older people living in the community. *British Medical Journal,* 2(316), 1348–1351.

Bidwell, S. (2004) Finding the evidence: resources and skills for locating information on clinical effectiveness. *Singapore Medical Journal,* 45(12), 567–572.

Blaxter, M. (1990) *Health and Lifestyles.* London: Routledge.

Boaden, R., Dusheiko, M., Gravelle, H., Parker, S., Pickard, S., Roland, M., Sargent, P. and Sheaff, R. (2006) *Evaluation of Evercare: Final Report.* University of Manchester: National Primary Care Research and Development Centre. Available from: www. population-health.manchester.ac.uk/primarycare/npcrdc-archive/archive/Publication Detail.cfm/ID/171.htm (accessed November 2014).

Bodenheimer, T., Lorig, K., Holman, H. and Grumbach, K. (2002) Patient self-management of chronic disease in primary care. *Journal of the American Medical Association (JAMA),* 288, 2469–2475.

Brehm, J. W. (1966) *A Theory of Psychological Reactance.* New York: Academic Press.

British Association of Occupational Therapists and College of Occupational Therapists (2014) *Long Term Conditions.* Available from: www.cot.co.uk/ot-helps-you/long-term-conditions (accessed September 2014).

British Association for Parenteral and Enteral Nutrition (BAPEN) (2003) *The 'MUST' Report. Nutritional Screening for Adults: A Multidisciplinary Responsibility.* Ed. M. Elia. Redditch: BAPEN.

British Association for Parenteral and Enteral Nutrition (BAPEN) (2011) *The 'MUST' Explanatory Booklet.* Rev. edn. Redditch: BAPEN.

British Association for Parenteral and Enteral Nutrition (BAPEN) (2014) *Malnutrition Matters: A Commitment to Act.* Redditch: BAPEN.

British Dietetic Association (BDA) (1997) *Obesity Treatment: Future Directions for the Contribution of Dieticians.* Position Paper. London: BDA.

British Heart Foundation (2014) *Cardiovascular Disease.* Available from: www.bhf.org.uk/ living_with_heart_conditions/understanding_heart_conditions/types_of_heart_ conditions/coronary_heart_disease.aspx (accessed July 2014).

British Lung Foundation (2014) *COPD.* Available from: www.lunguk.org/you-and-your-lungs/conditions-and-diseases/copd.htm (accessed July 2014).

British Medical Association (BMA) (2004) *Diabetes Mellitus: An Update for Healthcare Professionals.* London: BMA.

British Medical Association (BMA)/NHS Confederation (2003) *Investing in General Practice – The GMS Contract.* London: BMA.

British Medical Association (BMA)/NHS Employers (2012) *Quality and Outcomes Framework for 2012/2013.* London: General Practitioners Committee/NHS Employers.

British Medical Journal (BMJ) (2000) Patients as partners in managing chronic disease. *British Medical Journal,* 320, 526–527.

British Medical Journal (BMJ) Clinical Evidence (2014) *BMJ Clinical Evidence.* Available from: http://clinicalevidence.bmj.com/x/set/static/cms/about-us.html (accessed December 2014).

British Thoracic Society (BTS)/Scottish Intercollegiate Guidelines Network (SIGN) (2014) *British Guideline on the Management of Asthma*. Available from: www.sign.ac.uk/guidelines/fulltext/141/index.html (accessed October 2014).

Capital and Coast District Health Board (2008) *Long Term Conditions Management Framework*. Available from: www.ccdhb.org.nz/planning/ltc/complete_ltc_framework_web.pdf (accessed November 2014).

Carrier, J. A. K. (2014) *The Social Organisation of Practice Nurses' Knowledge Utilisation – An Ethnographic Study*. Cardiff University: unpublished PhD thesis.

Cavill, N., Hillsdon, M. and Anstiss, T. (2011) *Brief Interventions for Weight Management*. Oxford: National Obesity Observatory.

Centers for Disease Control and Prevention (CDCP) (2014) *Chronic Diseases and Health Promotion*. Available from: www.cdc.gov/chronicdisease/overview/index.htm (accessed November 2014).

Centre for Economic Policy Research (2008) *Does Unemployment Damage Your Health?* London: CEPR.

Centre for Reviews and Dissemination (CRD) (2008) *CRD Database*. Available from: www.crd.york.ac.uk/CRDWeb/ (accessed July 2008).

Centre for Reviews and Dissemination (CRD) (2009) *Systematic Reviews: CRD's Guidance for Undertaking Systematic Reviews in Health Care*. Available from: www.york.ac.uk/inst/crd/index_guidance.htm (accessed August 2014).

Centre for Workforce Intelligence (CfWI) (2012) *Workforce Risks and Opportunities Practice Nurses*. Surrey: CfWI.

Chowdhury, T. (2003) Preventing diabetes in south Asians: too little action and too late. *British Medical Journal*, 327(7423), 1059–1060.

Clinical Knowledge Summaries (CKS) (2010a) *Diabetes – Type 1*. Available from: http://cks.nice.org.uk/diabetes-type-1 (accessed August 2014).

Clinical Knowledge Summaries (CKS) (2010b) *Diabetes – Type 2*. Available from: http://cks.nice.org.uk/diabetes-type-2 (accessed August 2014).

Clinical Knowledge Summaries (CKS) (2010c) *Heart Failure*. Available from: http://cks.nice.org.uk/heart-failure-chronic (accessed July 2010).

Clinical Knowledge Summaries (CKS) (2011) *Chest Pain*. Available from: http://cks.nice.org.uk/chest-pain#!topicsummary (accessed August 2014).

Clinical Knowledge Summaries (CKS) (2013a) *Osteoporosis*. Available from: http://cks.nice.org.uk/osteoporosis-prevention-of-fragility-fractures (accessed October 2014).

Clinical Knowledge Summaries (CKS) (2013b) *Eczema*. Available from: http://cks.nice.org.uk/eczema-atopic (accessed October 2013).

Clinical Knowledge Summaries (CKS) (2013c) *Osteoarthritis*. Available from: www.nice.org.uk/guidance/cg177/chapter/1-recommendations#diagnosis-2 (accessed October 2014).

Clinical Knowledge Summaries (CKS) (2013d) *Rheumatoid Arthritis*. Available from: http://cks.nice.org.uk/rheumatoid-arthritis (accessed October 2014).

Clinical Knowledge Summaries (CKS) (2014a) *Angina*. Available from: http://cks.nice.org.uk/angina#!topicsummary (accessed September 2014).

Clinical Knowledge Summaries (CKS) (2014b) *Epilepsy*. Available from: http://cks.nice.org.uk/epilepsy (accessed November 2014).

Conner, M. and Norman, P. (2005) (eds) *Predicting Health Behaviour*, 2nd edn. Buckingham: Open University Press.

Connolly, M. and Boyd, M. A. (eds) ABCC New Zealand Study (2011) *Alleviating the Burden of Chronic Conditions in New Zealand*. Auckland: District Health Boards.

Corben, S. and Rosen, R. (2005) *Self-management for Long-term Conditions*. London: The King's Fund.

Coulter, A., Roberts, S. and Dixon, A. (2013) *Delivering Better Services for People with Long-Term Conditions: Building the House of Care*. London: The King's Fund.

Courtenay, M., Carey, N. and Stenner, K. (2009) Nurse prescriber-patient consultations: a case study in dermatology. *Journal of Advanced Nursing*, 65, 1207–1217.

Courtenay, M., Stenner, K. and Carey, N. (2010) The views of patients with diabetes about nurse prescribing. *Diabetic Medicine*, 27, 1049–1054.

Craig, P. (2002) The development of public health nursing. In Cowley, S. (ed.) *Public Health in Policy and Practice: A Sourcebook for Health Visitors and Community Nurses*. London: Bailliere Tindall.

Cullum, N. (2000) Users' guide to the nursing literature: an introduction. *Evidence Based Nursing*, 3(3), 71–72.

Dahlgren, G. and Whitehead, M. (1991) *Policies and Strategies to Promote Social Equity in Health*. Stockholm: Institute for Future Studies.

Department for Environment, Food and Rural Affairs (DEFRA) (2008) *Departmental Report*. Cm 7399. London: DEFRA.

Department of Health (DH) (1990) *General Medical Services Council – New GP Contract* London: HMSO.

Department of Health (DH) (1991) *Research for Health: A Research and Development Strategy for the NHS*. London: HMSO.

Department of Health (DH) (1992) *The Health of the Nation*. London: HMSO.

Department of Health (DH) (1997) *The New NHS: Modern, Dependable*. London: The Stationery Office.

Department of Health (DH) (1998) *A First Class Service: Quality in the New NHS*. London: HMSO.

Department of Health (DH) (1999) *Saving Lives: Our Healthier Nation*. London: Department of Health.

Department of Health (DH) (2000a) *National Service Framework for Coronary Heart Disease*. London: HMSO.

Department of Health (DH) (2000b) *The NHS Plan: A Plan for Investment, A Plan for Reform*. London: HMSO.

Department of Health (DH) (2000c) *Pharmacy in the Future*. London: HMSO.

Department of Health (DH) (2001) *The Expert Patient: A New Approach to Chronic Disease Management for the 21st Century*. London: Department of Health Publications.

Department of Health (DH) (2002a) *National Service Framework for Diabetes*. London: Department of Health Publications.

Department of Health (DH) (2002b) *Liberating the Talents*. London: Department of Health Publications.

Department of Health (DH) (2004a) *Chronic Disease Management*. London: Department of Health Publications.

Department of Health (DH) (2004b) *The NHS Improvement Plan: Putting People at the Heart of Public Services*. London: Department of Health Publications.

Department of Health (DH) (2005a) *Supporting People with Long Term Conditions. Liberating the Talents of Nurses who Care for People with Long Term Conditions*. London: Department of Health Publications.

Department of Health (DH) (2005b) *Supporting People with Long Term Conditions. An NHS Social Care Model to Support Local Innovation and Integration*. London: Department of Health Publications.

Department of Health (DH) (2005c) *National Service Framework for Long Term Conditions* Available from: www.dh.gov.uk/en/Publicationsandstatistics/Publications/Publications PolicyAndGuidance/DH_4105361 (accessed July 2014).

Department of Health (DH) (2006) *Our Health, Our Care, Our Say: A New Direction for Community Services*. London: Department of Health Publications.

Department of Health (DH) (2007a) *Long Term Conditions*. Available from: www.dh.gov.uk/en/Policyandguidance/Healthandsocialcaretopics/Longtermconditions/index.htm (accessed December 2008).

Department of Health (DH) (2007b) *National Stroke Strategy*. London: Department of Health.

Department of Health (DH) (2008a) *National Service Frameworks (NSFs.)* Available from: www.dh.gov.uk/en/ArchivedSections/Healthandsocialcaretopics/DH_4070951 (accessed December 2008).

Department of Health (DH) (2008b) *Raising the Profile of Long Term Conditions Care – A Compendium of Information*. London: Department of Health Publications.

Department of Health (DH) (2009) *Living Well with Dementia: A National Dementia Strategy*. London: Department of Health.

Department of Health (DH) (2012) *Long Term Conditions Compendium of Information*, 3rd edn. London: Department of Health. Available from: www.dh.gov.uk/publications (accessed August 2014).

Department of Health (DH) (2013a) *The Mandate – A Mandate from the Government to the NHS Commissioning Board April 2013 to March 2015*. Available from: http://webarchive.nationalarchives.gov.uk/20130503032958/http://mandate.dh.gov.uk/2012/11/13/nhs-mandate-published/ (accessed December 2008).

Department of Health (DH) (2013b) *Improving Quality of Life for People with Long Term Conditions*. London: Department of Health. Available from: www.gov.uk/government/policies/improving-quality-of-life-for-people-with-long-term-conditions (accessed July 2014).

Department of Health, Social Services and Public Safety (DHSSPSNI) (2005) *A Healthier Future – A Twenty Year Vision for Health and Well-being in Northern Ireland*. Available from: www.dhsspsni.gov.uk/healthyfuture-section2.pdf (accessed November 2014).

Department of Health, Social Services and Public Safety (DHSSPSNI) (2009) *Service Framework for Cardiovascular Health and Wellbeing*. Northern Ireland: Department of Health, Social Services and Public Safety.

Department of Health, Social Services and Public Safety (DHSSPSNI) (2011) *Service Framework for Mental Health and Wellbeing*. Northern Ireland: Department of Health, Social Services and Public Safety.

Department of Health, Social Services and Public Safety (DHSSPSNI) (2012a) *Living with Long Term Conditions – A Policy Framework*. Northern Ireland: Department of Health, Social Services and Public Safety.

Department of Health, Social Services and Public Safety (DHSSPSNI) (2012b) *Transforming Your Care*. Available from: www.dhsspsni.gov.uk/index/tyc.htm (accessed July 2014).

De Silva, D. (2011) *Helping People Help Themselves*. London: The Health Foundation.

Diabetes UK (2014) *Long Term Complications*. Available from: www.diabetes.org.uk/Guide-to-diabetes/Complications/Long_term_complications/ (accessed July 2014).

Diabetes UK, Department of Health, The Health Foundation and NHS Diabetes (2011) *Year of Care: Report of Findings from the Pilot Programme*. London: Diabetes UK, Department of Health, The Health Foundation, NHS Diabetes.

Dixon, A., Khachatryan, A., Wallace, A., Peckham, S., Boyce, T. and Gillam, S. (2011) *Impact of Quality and Outcomes Framework on Health Inequalities?* London: The King's Fund.

Donnelly, L. (2008) Don't treat the old and unhealthy, say doctors. *The Telegraph*. Available from: www.telegraph.co.uk (accessed July 2008).

Drennan, V. and Goodman, C. (2004) Nurse-led case management for older people with long-term conditions. *British Journal of Community Nursing*, 9(12), 527–533.

Eaton, S. (2012) We do it already ... don't we? In Department of Health, *Long Term Conditions: Developing a Cross-government Strategy*. London: Department of Health.

Eddy, D. M. (2005) Evidence-based medicine: a unified approach. *Health Affairs*, 24(1), 9–17.

meaningfulness of the patient-practitioner encounter. *Joanna Briggs Institute Database of Systematic Reviews*.

Reeves, D., Hann, M., Rick, J., Rowe, K., Small, N., Burt, J., Roland, M., Protheroe, J., Blakeman, T., Richardson, G., Kennedy, A. and Bower, P. (2014) Care plans and care planning in the management of long-term conditions in the UK. *British Journal of General Practice*. Available from: www.keele.ac.uk/pressreleases/2014/careplansandcareplanning inthemanagementoflong-termconditionsintheuk.html (accessed December 2014).

Renal Association (2007) *Stages of CKD (Chronic Kidney Disease)*. Available from: www.renal.org/eGFR/ckdstages.html (link no longer available).

Renal Asociation (2013) *2013 Guidelines*. Available from: www.renal.org/information-resources/the-uk-eckd-guide/ckd-stages#sthash.zVfInmWA.D56cN4yB.dpbs (accessed December 2014).

Renders, C. M., Valk, G. D., Griffin, S. J., Wagner, E. H., Eijk Van, J. T. and Assendelft, W. J. (2001) Interventions to improve the management of diabetes mellitus in primary care, outpatient and community settings. *Cochrane Database of Systematic Reviews*, Issue 2.

Rethink (2006) *Self-management*. Available from: www.rethink.org/recovery (accessed June 2014).

Riemsma, R. P., Kirwan, J. R., Taal, E. and Rasker, J. J. (2003) Patient education for adults with rheumatoid arthritis. *Cochrane Database of Systematic Reviews*, Issue 2.

Robb, G. and Seddon, M. (2006) Quality improvement in New Zealand healthcare. Part 6: keeping the patient front and centre to improve healthcare quality. *Journal of the New Zealand Medical Association*, 119, 1242.

Rollnick, S., Miller, W. and Butler, C. (2007) *Motivational Interviewing in Healthcare*. New York: Guilford Press.

Rosengren, D. B. (2009) *Building Motivational Interviewing Skills: A Practitioner Workbook*. New York: Guilford Press.

Ross, S., Curry, N. and Goodwin, N. (2011) *Case Management*. London: The King's Fund.

Roter, D. and Kinmonth, A. L. (2002) What is the evidence that increasing participation of individuals in self-management improves the process and outcomes of care? In Williams, R., Kinmonth, A. L., Wareham, N. and Herman, W. (eds) *The Evidence Base for Diabetes Care*. New York: Wiley.

Royal College of General Practitioners (RCGP) (2007) *The Primary Care Practice and Its Team. Information Sheet*. London: RCGP.

Royal College of Nursing (RCN) (2014) *Quality Improvement*. Available from: www.rcn.org.uk/development/practice/clinical_governance/quality_improvement (accessed November 2014).

Royal Pharmaceutical Society of Great Britain and the British Medical Association (BMA) (2000) *Teamworking in Primary Healthcare – Final Report*. London: Royal Pharmaceutical Society of Great Britain and BMA.

Rubak, S., Sandboek, A., Lauritzen, T. and Christensen, B. (2005) Motivational interviewing: a systematic review and meta-analysis. *British Journal of General Practice*, 55, 305–312.

Rycroft-Malone, J., Fontenla, M., Seers, K. and Bick, D. (2009) Protocol-based care: the standardisation of decision-making? *Journal of Clinical Nursing*, 18, 1490–1500.

Sackett, D. L., Rosenberg, W. M., Muir Gray, J. A., Haynes, R. B. and Richardson, W. S. (1996) Evidence-based medicine: what it is and what it isn't. *British Medical Journal*, 312, 71–72.

Sackett, D. L., Straus, S. E., Richardson, W. S., Rosenberg, W. and Haynes, R. B. (2000) *Evidence Based Medicine: How to Practice and Teach EBM*, 2nd edn. Edinburgh: Churchill-Livingstone.

Schumacher, J. A. and Madson, M. B. (2014) *Fundamentals of Motivational Interviewing: Tips and Strategies for Addressing Common Clinical Challenges*. New York: Oxford University Press.

Shumaker, S. A., Ockene, J. K. and Riekert, K. A. (eds) (2009) *The Handbook of Health Behavior Change*, 3rd edn. New York: Springer.

Scott, A., Sivey, P., Ait Ouakrim, D., Willenberg, L., Naccarella, L., Furler, J. and Young, D. (2011) The effect of financial incentives on the quality of health care provided by primary care physicians. *Cochrane Database of Systematic Reviews*, Issue 9.

Scottish Government (2008) *Better Health, Better Care: Action Plan. What It Means for You*. Edinburgh: Scottish Government.

Scottish Government (2009a) *Better Heart Disease and Stroke Care Action Plan*. Edinburgh: Scottish Government.

Scottish Government (2009b) *Improving Health and Wellbeing of People with Long Term Conditions: A National Action Plan*. Edinburgh: Scottish Government.

Scottish Intercollegiate Guidelines Network (SIGN) (2006) *Diagnosis and Management of Peripheral Arterial Disease*. Available from: www.sign.ac.uk/pdf/sign89.pdf (accessed July 2008).

Scottish Intercollegiate Guidelines Network (SIGN) (2008) *Diagnosis and Management of Chronic Kidney Disease*. Available from: www.renal.org/pages/media/Guidelines/sign103.pdf (accessed July 2008).

Sheehy, C., Murphy, E. and Barry, M. (2006) Depression in rheumatoid arthritis: underscoring the problem. *Rheumatolgy*, 45, 1325–1327.

Singh, D. and Ham, C. (2006) *Improving Care for People with Long-Term Conditions: A Review of UK and International Frameworks*. University of Birmingham: NHS Institute for Innovation and Improvement and Health Services Management Centre.

South Canterbury District Health Board (2009) *A Strategic Framework for the Prevention and Management of Long Term Conditions*. Available from: www.scdhb.health.nz/uploads/File/Key_documents/Chronic%20Conditions%20Framework%20finalJudy June1209.pdf (accessed November 2014).

Stanford University School of Medicine Patient Education Research Centre (2008) *Chronic Disease Self-Management Program*. Available from: http://patienteducation.stanford.edu/programs/cdsmp.html (accessed November 2014).

Steinberg, E. and Luce, B. (2005). Evidence based? Caveat emptor! *Health Affairs*, 24(1), 80–92.

Stenner, K. and Courtenay, M. (2008) The benefits of nurse prescribing according to nurses prescribing for patients in pain. *Journal of Advanced Nursing*, 63, 27–35.

Stenner, K., Carey, N. and Courtenay, M. (2010) Implementing nurse prescribing: a case study in diabetes. *Journal of Advanced Nursing*, 66(3), 522–531.

Stokes, T., Shaw, E. J., Camosso-Stefinovic, J., Baker, R., Baker, G. A. and Jacoby, A. (2007) Self-management education for children with epilepsy. *Cochrane Database of Systematic Reviews*, Issue 2.

Stratton, R. J., Green, C. J. and Elia, M. (2003). *Disease-Related Malnutrition: An Evidence Based Approach to Treatment*. Wallingford: CABI Publishing.

Telecare Services Association (2013) *What is Telecare/Telehealth?* Available from: www.telecare.org.uk/consumer-services/what-is-telecare (accessed December 2014).

The Cochrane Collaboration (2008) *Archie Cochrane: The Name Behind the Cochrane Collaboration*. Available from: www.cochrane.org/docs/archieco.htm (accessed July 2014).

The Psoriasis Association (2014) *About Psoriasis*. Available from: www.psoriasis-association.org.uk/pages/view/about-psoriasis (accessed November 2014).

The Stroke Association (2014) *When A Stroke Happens*. Available from: www.stroke.org.uk/factsheet/when-stroke-happens (accessed December 2014).

Thomas, B. and Bishop, J. (2007) *The Manual of Dietetic Practice*, 4th edn. Oxford: Blackwell.

Thompson, H. and Ryan, A. (2008) A review of the psychosocial consequences of stroke and their impact on spousal relationships. *British Journal of Neuroscience Nursing*, 4(4), 177–184.

Timmermans, S. and Berg, M. (2003) *The Gold Standard – The Challenge of Evidence-based Medicine and Standardization in Health Care*. Philadelphia, PA: Temple University Press.

Toelle, B. G. and Ram, F. S. F. (2004) Written individualised management plans for asthma in children and adults. *Cochrane Database of Systematic Reviews*, Issue 1.

Tudor-Hart, J. (1971) 'The Inverse Care Law'. *The Lancet*, 27 February, 405–412.

Turnock, A. C., Walters, E. H., Walters, J. A. E. and Wood-Baker, R. (2005) Action plans for chronic obstructive pulmonary disease. *Cochrane Database of Systematic Reviews*, Issue 4.

Uchino, B. N. (2006) Social support and health: a review of physiological processes potentially underlying links to disease outcomes. *Journal of Behavioral Medicine*, 29, 377–387.

UNICEF (2007) *The State of the World's Children, 2008. Child Survival*. New York: UNICEF.

van Dam, H. A., van der Horst, F., van den Borne, B., Ryckman, R. and Crebolder, H. (2003) Provider-patient interaction in diabetes care: effects on patient self-care outcomes – a systematic review. *Patient Education and Counselling*, 51(1), 17–28.

Wagner, E. H. (1998) Chronic disease management: what will it take to improve care for chronic illness? *Effective Clinical Practice*, 1, 2–4.

Wagner, E. H., Austin, B. T., Davis, C., Hindmarsh, M., Schaefer, J. and Bonomi, A. (2001) Improving chronic illness care: translating evidence into action. *Health Affairs*, 20(6), 64–78.

Wales Audit Office (2014) *The Management of Chronic Conditions in Wales*. Cardiff: Wales Audit Office.

Walters, J., Turnock, A., Walters, H. and Wood-Baker, R. (2010) Action plans with limited patient education only for exacerbations of chronic obstructive pulmonary disease. *Cochrane Database of Systematic Reviews*, Issue 5.

Welsh Assembly Government (WAG) (2001) *Improving Health in Wales: A Plan for the NHS with its Partners*. Cardiff: WAG.

Welsh Assembly Government (WAG) (2005) *Designed for Life – A World Class Health Service for Wales*. Cardiff: WAG.

Welsh Assembly Government (WAG) (2007a) *Designed to Tackle Renal Disease in Wales: A National Service Framework*. Cardiff: WAG.

Welsh Assembly Government (WAG) (2007b) *Designed to Improve Health and the Management of Chronic Conditions in Wales: An Integrated Model and Framework for Action*. Cardiff: WAG.

Welsh Assembly Government (WAG)/National Public Health Service Wales (NPHS) (2005) *A Profile of Long Term and Chronic Conditions in Wales*. Cardiff: WAG.

Welsh Government (WG) (2006) *National Service Framework for Older People*. Cardiff: Welsh Government.

Welsh Government (WG) (2010) *Setting the Direction*. Cardiff: Welsh Government.

Welsh Government (WG) (2012) *Together for Health*. Cardiff: Welsh Government.

Welsh Government (WG) (2013a) *Welsh Health Survey Knowledge and Analytical Services*. Cardiff: Welsh Government. Available from: http://wales.gov.uk/statistics-and-research/welsh-health-survey/?lang=en (accessed September 2014).

Welsh Government (WG) (2013b) *Together for Health – A Diabetes Delivery Plan*. Cardiff: Welsh Government.

Welsh Government (WG) (2014a) *Together for Health – A Respiratory Health Delivery Plan*. Cardiff: Welsh Government.

Welsh Government (WG) (2014b) *Together for Health – Heart Disease Delivery Plan*. Cardiff: Welsh Government.

While, A. (2007) Lessons from the Evercare evaluation. *British Journal of Community Nursing*, 12(1), 46.

Wilson, P. M. (2005) Long-term conditions: making sense of the current policy agenda. *British Journal of Community Nursing*, 10(12), 544–552.

Wilson, T., Buck, D. and Ham, C. (2005) Rising to the challenge: will the NHS support people with long term conditions? *British Medical Journal*, 330, 657–661.

World Health Organisation (WHO) (1978) *The Declaration of Alma Ata. International Conference on Primary Health Care*. Geneva: WHO.

World Health Organisation (WHO) (1986) *Ottawa Charter for Health Promotion*. Ottawa: WHO.

World Health Organisation (WHO) (1990) *Cancer Plan Relief and Palliative Care*. Geneva: WHO.

World Health Organisation (WHO) (1991) *Community Involvement in Health Development: Challenging Health Services*. Geneva: WHO.

World Health Organisation (WHO) (1998) *Obesity: Preventing and Managing the Global Epidemic*. Geneva: WHO.

World Health Organisation (WHO) (2002a) *The Impact of Chronic Disease in New Zealand*. Available from: www.who.int/chp/chronic_disease_report/media/impact/new_zealand.pdf (accessed December 2014).

World Health Organisation (WHO) (2002b) *Innovative Care for Chronic Conditions*. Available from: www.who.int/diabetes/publications/icccreport/en/ (accessed December 2014).

World Health Organization (WHO) (2006a) *COPD: Burden*. Available from: www.who.int/respiratory/copd/burden/en/index.htm (accessed December 2014).

World Health Organization (WHO) (2006b) *Definition and Diagnosis of Diabetes Mellitus and Intermediate Hyperglycaemia*. Available from: www.who.int/diabetes/publications/Definition%20and%20diagnosis%20of%20diabetes_new.pdf (accessed December 2014).

World Health Organisation (WHO) (2009) *2008–2013 Action Plan for the Global Strategy for the Prevention and Control of Noncommunicable Diseases*. Geneva: WHO.

World Health Organisation (WHO) (2010) *Global Status Report on Noncommunicable Diseases 2010*. Geneva: WHO. Available from: www.who.int/nmh/publications/ncd_report2010/en/ (accessed May 2014).

World Health Organisation (WHO) (2011) *Use of Glycated Haemoglobin (HbA1c) in the Diagnosis of Diabetes Mellitus*. Available from: www.who.int/diabetes/publications/report-hba1c_2011.pdf (accessed September 2014).

World Health Organisation (WHO) (2013) *Global Action Plan for the Prevention and Control of Noncommunicable Diseases 2013–2020*. Available from: http://apps.who.int/iris/bitstream/10665/94384/1/9789241506236_eng.pdf?ua=1 (accessed July 2014).

World Health Organisation (WHO) (2014a) *Chronic Diseases and Health Promotion*. Available from: www.who.int/chp/en/ (accessed July 2014).

World Health Organisation (WHO) (2014b) *Note for the Media – WHO Highlights Need for Countries to Scale up Action on Noncommunicable Diseases*. Available from: www.who.int/mediacentre/news/notes/2014/action-on-ncds/en/ (accessed July 2014).

# Index